Sleep

Your Questions Answered

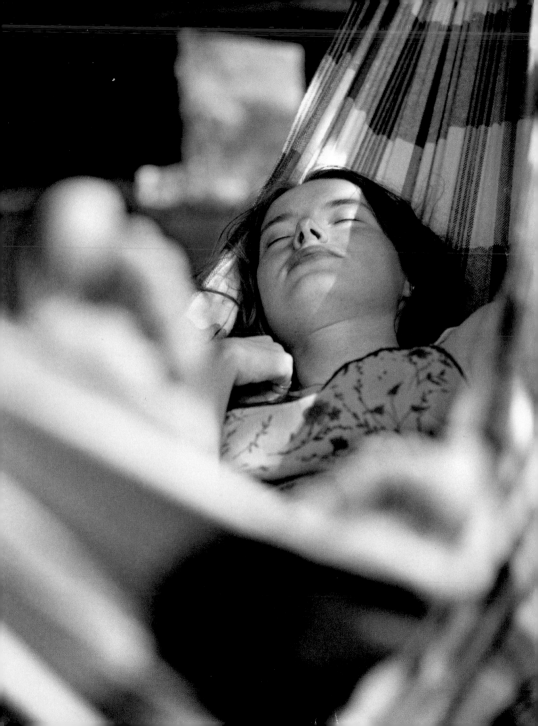

Sleep

Your Questions Answered

Renata L. Riha, MD

US medical editor: Anne Helena Rennes, MD

LONDON, NEW YORK, MUNICH, MELBOURNE, DELHI

DORLING KINDERSLEY
Editor Tom Broder
Senior Art Editor Nicola Rodway
US Senior Editor Jill Hamilton
Executive Managing Editor Adèle Hayward
Managing Art Editor Nick Harris
DTP Designer Traci Salter
Production Controller Clara Mclean
Art Director Peter Luff
Publisher Corinne Roberts

DK INDIA
Senior Editor Dipali Singh
Project Editor Rohan Sinha
Editors Ankush Saikia, Aakriti Singhal
Project Designer Romi Chakraborty
DTP Coordinator Pankaj Sharma
DTP Designer Balwant Singh, Sunil Sharma
Head of Publishing Aparna Sharma

Edited for Dorling Kindersley by
Philip Morgan

First American Edition, 2007

Published in the United States by DK Publishing
375 Hudson Street, New York, New York 10014

07 08 09 10 11   10 9 8 7 6 5 4 3 2 1
SD244—April, 2007

Published in Great Britain by Dorling Kindersley Limited.

A catalog record for this book is available from the Library of Congress.

ISBN: 978-0-7566-2618-1

DK books are available at special discounts when purchased in bulk for sales promotions, premiums, fund-raising, or educational use. For details, contact: DK Publishing Special Markets, 375 Hudson Street, New York, New York 10014 or SpecialSales@dk.com.

Printed and bound in Singapore by Tien Wah Press

Discover more at www.dk.com

Foreword

Everyone knows what sleep is but it is very difficult to define. We spend a third of our lives asleep and a good night's sleep is integral to our health and well-being. Sleep disorders are common within our society and contribute to impaired academic and job performance. They can result in accidents at work and while driving, thereby raising significant public health issues. They can lead to impaired mood and they can affect social adjustment. Relationships can be severely affected by the disordered sleep of a bed partner. Sleep disorders can also lead to or worsen underlying medical and psychiatric problems.

This book attempts to describe the basic processes of sleep and the disorders associated with it. Sleep disorders are outlined and treatments discussed. Practical suggestions for getting a good night's sleep and dealing with common problems that affect sleep throughout life are also presented. If you ever have any concerns at all about your health, lifestyle, or sleep, you should consult a professional. I hope this book will help you know what questions to ask, and what to expect. Sleep well!

Dr. Renata L. Riha

Contents

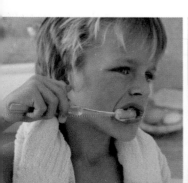
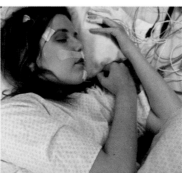
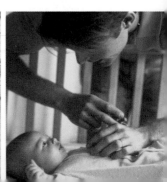

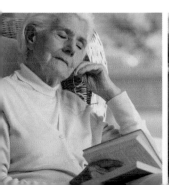
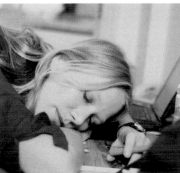
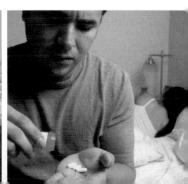

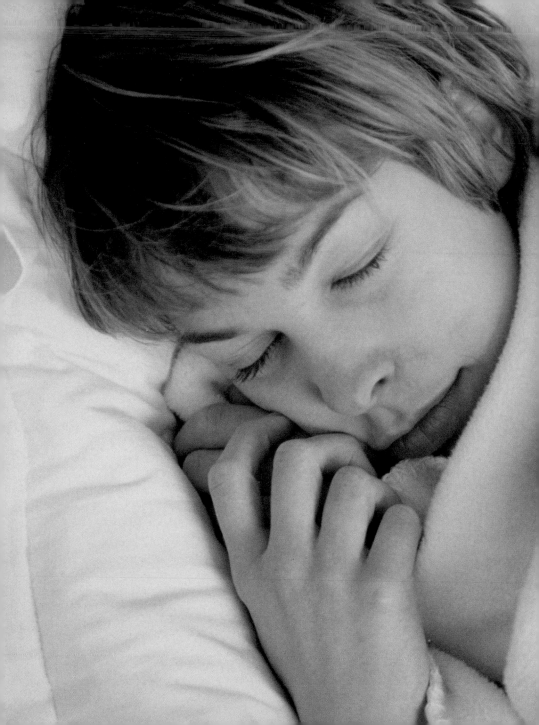

Understanding sleep

We spend about a third of our lives asleep, yet we are still not sure why we sleep. What we do know is that we need enough good-quality sleep to function well while we are awake. The type of sleep we experience, and our sleep requirements, change over time, depending on our activity levels, our health, and our environment. This chapter explores some key aspects of normal sleep in adults.

The rhythms of sleep

Q What is sleep?

Everyone knows what sleep is, but would find it difficult to define. Perhaps the scientist Robert McNish summed it up best when he wrote in *The Philosophy of Sleep* (1834): "Sleep is the intermediate state between wakefulness and death; wakefulness being regarded as the active state of all the animal and intellectual functions, and death as that of their total suspension." During sleep, our senses are disengaged and we are temporarily unresponsive to our environment. Sleep involves processes affecting both our behavior and our physiology (the way the body works).

Q Why do we need sleep?

Sleep is important to health, and insufficient sleep can lead to problems with various body systems, including the immune system, the heart and circulatory system, and hormone secretion. Also, poor-quality or insufficient sleep can lead to impairment of daytime functioning, excessive daytime sleepiness, and problems with memory.

Q How much do we know about sleep?

The study of sleep is an evolving science. We know a lot about many disorders of sleep but not enough about others. Answers to even the most common questions about sleep are not always simple or straightforward, and sometimes there is no answer at all. Studies in sleep and sleep disorders are a relatively new area of research compared with many other areas of human health.

Q How long has sleep been studied?

The study of sleep and sleep disorders is a relatively new discipline in science and medicine. In 1875, differences in the brain activity of sleeping and awake dogs were studied using electroencephalograms (EEGs), which recorded electrical impulses in the brain. In 1880, the classic features of narcolepsy (a sleep disorder characterized by excessive daytime sleepiness; see p55) were described. Specific sleep disorders were identified as interest in sleep, and the method of documentation of these disorders—the polysomnogram— evolved. The first narcolepsy clinics were set up in 1964, and the use of continuous positive airway pressure (CPAP) for the treatment of sleep apnea (see pp58–61) was introduced in 1981.

WHAT ARE CIRCADIAN RHYTHMS?

Circadian rhythms are the "clocks" of our internal mechanism that determine the phases of our cellular and organ activity over a 24-hour period. The word circadian means "about a day." Circadian rhythms affect body temperature, organ function, secretion of hormones such as cortisol (the primary stress hormone), and sleep. Each rhythm affects the others. In an environment with no time cues (such as light, clocks, calendars) our body clock completes a cycle that is slightly longer than the natural day—about 24 hours and 42 minutes, rather than exactly 24 hours.

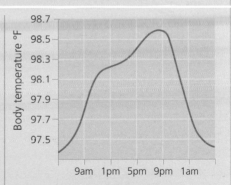

BODY TEMPERATURE AND SLEEP *Our body's circadian rhythms dictate the rise and fall of our internal temperature over the course of a day. We are most likely to fall asleep when our body temperature is in the downward phase.*

Q What is the sleep-wake cycle?

The sleep-wake cycle is the alternation between the states of being awake and being asleep. One theory of sleep states that the amount of sleep we experience depends on the length of time we are awake prior to sleep. So, the longer you are awake and the more tired and sleepy you become, the greater the urge for you to fall asleep and the longer you are likely to sleep in order for your body to attain "normal function" again. Some researchers believe there is a separate sleep-wake cycle that runs on its own rhythm but also interacts with the circadian rhythm. Many other theories have been developed in order to define how and why we sleep and what the basic drives to sleep are.

Q What role does cortisol play in the sleep-wake cycle?

Cortisol is the "stress response" hormone of the body. It has a marked circadian rhythm, and levels in the blood will vary during the day and night. Cortisol levels are at their lowest during slow wave sleep (see p17) at night. The highest cortisol levels are in the early morning before sunrise and awakening. This means that your body is prepared to be fully active when you get up.

Q What role does body temperature play in regulating sleep?

Sleep onset is likeliest to occur in the downward phase of the temperature cycle (see p11). In other words, we are most likely to sleep when our body temperature is falling. A secondary peak in sleepiness occurs in the afternoon and corresponds to afternoon napping. Sleep stops as the body temperature curve rises.

Q Is environmental temperature important in sleep?

It is usually more conducive to sleep in a slightly cooler rather than warmer environment, since this matches the dip in core body temperature that occurs during sleep. Extremes of temperature (hot or cold) disrupt sleep.

Q Which parts of the brain are involved in sleep?

The most important part of the brain involved in the coordination of the sleep process is called the reticular activating system (RAS). It is composed of a large number of nerve cells throughout the brain and is responsible for regulating wakefulness. When the RAS neurons switch off, alertness is reduced. There is a significant and continuous interplay between the RAS and other sleep-regulating areas in the brain. These include the thalamus, medulla oblongata, hypothalamus, pons, midbrain, spinal cord, pineal gland, raphe nuclei, basal forebrain, hippocampus, and suprachiasmatic nucleus.

Q Why is the suprachiasmatic nucleus important?

The suprachiasmatic nucleus is a system of nerve cells responsible for the circadian rhythm. It is strongly affected by light and promotes wakefulness, as shown by the high firing rate of the neurons in the day and low firing rate at night. Neurons from the suprachiasmatic nucleus project to many areas of the brain including the thalamus The suprachiasmatic nucleus also regulates the timing of melatonin secretion from the pineal gland (see p18).

Q What role do light and darkness play in regulating sleep?

Light activates special receptor cells at the back of the eye (retina), which in turn affect the suprachiasmatic nucleus. This has links to other parts of the brain that regulate sleep and wakefulness, including the pineal gland, which produces melatonin. Exposure to light increases wakefulness while darkness has the opposite effect. Light is thus important to the regulation of sleep and wakefulness and helps keep our circadian rhythm on track. Light is an effective cue for wakefulness in all humans, except those who lack light receptors in the eyes (certain forms of profound blindness).

HOW IS SLEEP MEASURED AND RECORDED?

Sleep doctors, sleep technologists, and sleep researchers use a system called polysomnography (PSG) to record a person's sleep, to diagnose many sleep disorders, and to investigate the differences between normal and abnormal sleep. The PSG is usually performed in a sleep laboratory, which can be part of a hospital or university research setting.

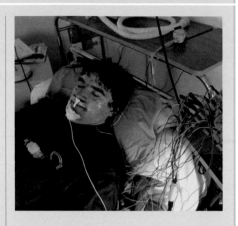

Sophisticated equipment is used to collect signals from a sleeping person. An electroencephalogram (EEG) records brain wave activity. An electro-oculogram (EOG) records the activity of the eyes and an electromyogram (EMG) records activity in muscles. Other equipment collects signals related to breathing (respiration), and records airflow through the nose and mouth, respiratory effort, movement, and oxygen and carbon dioxide levels. An electrocardiogram (ECG) monitors heart rate and rhythm. Electrodes placed on the muscles of the shins, together with a body position sensor around the waist, record body movement and leg or arm movement.

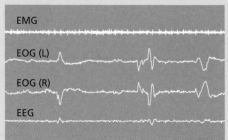

MONITORING YOUR SLEEP *This recording of REM sleep shows the typical rapid eye movements (EOG), low muscle tone (EMG), and the characteristic brain wave pattern (EEG). REM sleep is distinct from NREM sleep in that we have an "active mind inside a paralyzed body." We often wake up from REM sleep, or just after it in the morning.*

The states of sleep

Q Are there different states of sleep?

There are two states of normal human sleep: nonrapid eye movement sleep, or NREM sleep, and rapid eye movement sleep, or REM sleep. NREM and REM sleep usually alternate in cyclically with each other. Under normal circumstances, you enter sleep through NREM sleep and this cycles with REM sleep at about 90–110-minute intervals. Young adults usually experience 4 to 5 REM periods throughout the time they are asleep.

Q What exactly is NREM sleep?

NREM sleep comprises light sleep and also slow wave sleep. By convention, NREM sleep is subdivided into 4 stages. Stages 1 and 2 are considered to be light sleep and stages 3 and 4 are called slow wave sleep. The 4 stages of NREM sleep parallel the depth of sleep. You are therefore most likely to waken easily in stage 1 and be very difficult to waken in stage 4 sleep. The best way to think of NREM sleep is as "a relatively inactive yet actively regulating brain in a movable body."

Q What exactly is REM sleep?

During REM sleep we have significant brain activity along with muscle atonia, which means that our muscles are effectively paralyzed, except for the muscles that move the eyes, the diaphragm (for breathing), and the heart. During REM sleep we experience episodic bursts of rapid eye movements. This is the period when we experience dreams. If woken from this stage of sleep, you are likely to have vivid dream recall about 80 percent of the time. The best way to think of REM sleep is as "a highly activated brain in a paralyzed body."

Q Is it normal to enter sleep through REM sleep?

Apart from circumstances such as "catch up" sleep after sleep deprivation, it is abnormal for an adult to enter sleep through REM sleep. But it is normal for infants up to the age of 3 months or so to have sleep-onset REM (also called active sleep). Between 3 and 6 months, NREM sleep (or inactive sleep) in infants becomes clearly demarcated.

Q What are the different stages of sleep in adults?

Sleep occurs in cycles. The first cycle begins with stage 1 NREM sleep, when it is easy to wake someone. Stage 2 NREM sleep has a higher arousal threshold. This stage lasts about 10–25 minutes. Stages 3 and 4 of NREM sleep are characterized by slow wave sleep, which takes up about 20–40 minutes in the first sleep cycle. Body movement and lightening of sleep occurs within about 5–10 minutes of stage 2 prior to going into the first episode of REM sleep of the night. This first period of REM sleep usually lasts for 1–5 minutes.

Q How long do the sleep cycles last?

NREM and REM stages of sleep alternate throughout the night in a circadian rhythm. In adults, the average duration of the first sleep cycle of the night is 70–100 minutes and later cycles last about 90–120 minutes. Slow wave sleep is dominant in the first third of the night and REM sleep is dominant in the last third. This is why we generally wake up from a dream or just after a dream in the morning.

Q What determines how much sleep I get?

The amount of NREM sleep depends on the initiation of sleep, how long you have been awake, and the duration of sleep. The amount of REM sleep is linked to the body clock and to circadian changes in body temperature. The length of NREM and REM sleep also change with age.

Q What happens during slow wave sleep?

During slow wave sleep, there is an increased secretion of growth hormone with about 70 percent of this hormone being produced during this stage. Slow wave sleep occurs in greater amounts during phases of growth (childhood into early adulthood), pregnancy, and breast-feeding (because of increased levels of the hormone prolactin) and also during illness and states of general inflammation (due to increased amounts of inflammatory molecules called cytokines). As slow wave sleep decreases with age, the amount of growth hormone secreted also declines. As our levels of growth hormone decline, there is an increase in our tendency to put on fat tissue, lose muscle mass and strength, and lose our capacity for vigorous exercise.

Q Does the time I go to sleep make a difference to the type of sleep I have?

If you regularly go to sleep late and wake up late—for example, 3–11am—the proportion and cycling of REM and NREM sleep will be normal. However, if you are sleep-deprived, both REM and NREM sleep are increased.

Q What are sleep starts?

On falling asleep, many people can experience a sudden jerking movement of the body that they find uncomfortable. This sensation can be associated with vivid imagery, such as a sensation of falling. This is an entirely normal phenomenon. It is called hypnic myoclonia, or sleep starts. Sleep starts can increase in frequency or intensity in times of stress or with irregular sleep-wake schedules. It is generally thought that sleep starts occur because we enter sleep through REM sleep, which is what happens in infancy.

Chemicals involved in sleep

Q What is melatonin?

Melatonin is a hormone produced by the pineal gland and has an important role in circadian rhythms. The daily rhythm of melatonin secretion is controlled by a built-in, free-running pacemaker, the suprachiasmatic nucleus (see p13), and is synthesized from the amino acid tryptophan. Melatonin synthesis is controlled by exposure to cycles of light and dark, and occurs independently of sleep.

Q What part does melatonin play in regulating sleep?

Melatonin promotes sleep and its secretion increases soon after the onset of darkness, helping to keep us asleep at night. Melatonin production usually peaks between midnight and 2am, then starts to fall and is low during the day. It also helps reduce core body temperature, which helps induce sleep. However, sleep is possible even when melatonin levels are low. People who have their pineal gland removed have only minimal disruption in sleep.

Q Does melatonin have any other effects on the body?

Laboratory experiments have shown that melatonin has antioxidant effects and suppresses the growth of some cancer cells. Laboratory findings also show it has anti-inflammatory effects. When melatonin is administered as a drug it has been shown to decrease levels of the female hormones progesterone and estradiol. It also enhances the secretion of prolactin (hormone produced by the pituitary gland). Melatonin may reduce the sensitivity of the body to insulin, which can raise blood sugar levels.

OTHER CHEMICALS INVOLVED IN SLEEP

A large number of neurotransmitters and hormones regulate the sleep-wake process in the brain and nervous system. Their major functions are listed below.

Norepinephrine/ Epinephrine	The "fight-or-flight" chemicals. These stimulate, enhance, or prolong a waking, attentive, and aroused state.
Dopamine	Arouses the cerebral cortex (gray matter); involved in the regulation of movement and responsiveness.
Acetylcholine	Activates the cerebral cortex; increases vigilance. Levels are highest when awake and in REM sleep.
Histamine	Activates cerebral cortex during wakefulness.
Hypocretin (Orexin)	Promotes wakefulness and prevents sleep, including REM sleep. Stimulates energy metabolism and regulates appetite.
Glutamate	Stimulates the central nervous system and activates the cerebral cortex. Critical to wakefulness.
GABA (gamma amino butyric acid)	Inhibits wakefulness. Sleep-inducing drugs enhance the action of GABA to cause sleepiness and drowsiness.
Galanin	Inhibits wakefulness.
Adenosine	Induces sleep and is blocked by caffeine. Levels build up during the day and drop during sleep.
Serotonin	Has a tranquilizing effect. May prepare brain and body for slow wave sleep by reducing the body's activating systems.
Insulin	Accumulates during active waking periods with food intake and can lead to induction of sleep subsequently.

Other chemicals that work together to regulate sleep include cytokines, prostaglandin D2, growth hormone releasing factor, opiate peptides, bombesin, and cholecystokinin.

Myth "Everyone needs about 8 hours of sleep every night"

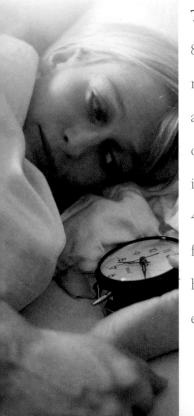

Truth An adult requires an average of 7.5–8.5 hours of sleep every night. However, this requirement varies widely between individuals and depends on age, genetics, and the amount of physical and mental activity. In very rare instances, some people can get by with just 4 hours of sleep (as Napoleon Bonaparte famously did), whereas some of us need 9–10 hours of sleep a day to function properly (for example, Albert Einstein).

Amount of sleep

Q What determines how much sleep I need?

Our sleep requirement is determined by a number of factors, including the amount of time spent awake, genetic factors, our age, and our circadian rhythm which initiates sleep. All of these factors vary on an individual basis, and explain why some people need more sleep than others and why these requirements can change with age.

Q How does age and aging affect sleep needs?

Newborns spend more than half their time asleep. Sleep needs decline over the first 5 years, again during the teenage years, and, finally, after the fifth decade. Sleep patterns also vary significantly. Infants can go from being awake straight into REM sleep, and their NREM–REM cycle is about 50–60 minutes. Children have the greatest percentage of slow wave sleep, which decreases by up to 40 percent between the ages of 10 and 20. Teens spend about 20–25 percent of sleep time in REM sleep. In old age, slow wave sleep may be absent, especially in men.

Q What is the difference between "night owls" and "early birds"?

"Night owls" refers to those who have a natural predisposition to staying up late and functioning well later in the day. "Early birds," on the other hand, get to bed early, wake early, and tend do their best work in the mornings. The vast majority of people fall between these two extremes. These differences are genetic and are caused by the circadian clock genes. Small mutations in one, some, or all of them may produce differences in the timing of our sleep. Subtle changes in the clock genes may have helped human beings adapt successfully to life in different environments with different levels of light.

Night owls and early birds

The following questionnaire is based on a longer questionnaire first published in 1976 and known as the Horne–Ostberg test. It explores whether you have a tendency to function better toward the end of a 24-hour day or at the beginning of one. Consider each question and choose the one response that best describes you. When you have answered all the questions, add up the score for each response. The final score will give you some indication of whether you are more of an "evening" person or a "morning" person.

Breakfast: how is your appetite in the first half hour after you wake up in the morning?
a) Very poor ①
b) Fairly poor ②
c) Fairly good ③
d) Very good ④

How do you feel for the first half hour after you wake up in the morning?
a) Very tired ①
b) Fairly tired ②
c) Fairly refreshed ③
d) Very refreshed ④

When you have no commitments the next day, at what time do you go to bed compared to your usual bedtime?
a) Seldom or never later ④
b) Less than 1 hour later ③
c) 1–2 hours later ②
d) More than 2 hours later ①

You are starting a new fitness regime. A friend suggests joining his fitness class between 7am and 8am. How do you think you'd perform?
a) Would be in good form ④
b) Would be in reasonable form ③
c) Would find it difficult ②
d) Would find it very difficult ①

At what time in the evening do you feel tired and in need of sleep?
a) 8pm–9pm ⑤
b) 9pm–10:15pm ④
c) 10:15pm–12:45am ③
d) 12:45am–2am ②
e) 2am–3am ①

If you went to bed at 11pm, how tired would you be?
a) Not at all tired ⓪
b) A little tired ②
c) Fairly tired ③
d) Very tired ⑤

One night you have to stay awake between 4am and 6am. You have no commitments the next day. Which suits you best?
a) Not to go to bed until 6am ①
b) Nap before 4am and after 6am ②
c) Sleep before 4am and nap after 6am ③
d) Sleep before 4am and remain awake after 6am ④

At what time of day do you feel your best?
a) Midnight–5am ①
b) 5am–9am ⑤
c) 9am–11am ④
d) 11am–5pm ③
e) 5pm–10pm ②
f) 10pm–midnight ①

Do you think of yourself as a morning or evening person?
a) Morning type ⑥
b) More morning than evening ④
c) More evening than morning ②
d) Evening type ⓪

Suppose that you can choose your own work hours, but had to work 5 hours in a day. When would you like to START your working day?
a) Midnight–5am ①
b) 3am–8am ⑤
c) 8am–10am ④
d) 10am–2pm ③
e) 2pm–4pm ②
f) 4pm–midnight ①

Scoring: To find out how much of a night owl or an early bird you are, add up the number of circled points that you scored for each answer. The maximum number of points you can get from this questionnaire is 46 and the minimum is 8. The higher your score, the more of an early bird you are. The lower your score, the more of a night owl you are, and you probably function better in the evenings. The majority of people come somewhere between these two extremes.

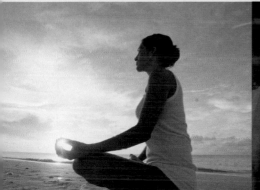

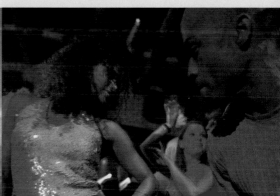

Dreams and dreaming

Q **What is dreaming?**

Dreaming, like sleep, is hard to define and some scientists prefer to use the term "sleep mentation," which means all the perceptions, emotions, and thoughts experienced during sleep (or its processes). Dreaming occurs mostly during REM sleep but can also occur in NREM sleep.

Q **Why do we dream?**

The purpose of dreaming is currently unknown. Physiological theories give it no real importance, while psychoanalytic theories hold the opposite view. What is known is that certain medications can intensify dreams or lead to nightmares, and that mood is affected by the type of dream or the sleep disturbance it causes. Dreaming is also believed by some to consolidate memory (see p45).

Q **What is the difference between REM and NREM dreams?**

REM dreams generally tend to be bizarre, vivid, and emotional, and are usually better recalled than NREM dreams, which are considered to be more thoughtlike, although not much may be remembered of them. Dream reports are more common from both of these states of sleep the later in the night a person is awakened.

Q **I don't dream—is this normal?**

Everybody dreams unless there has been significant damage to the brain. Some people are just better at remembering their dreams than others.

Q **What is lucid dreaming?**

Lucid dreaming is the conscious perception of one's dream, sometimes enabling direct control over the content of the dreams. They are not nightmares. Some psychiatrists use the technique of lucid dreaming in therapy.

Q What are nightmares?

We've all had nightmares. They are very common in both adults and children. Nightmares are emotionally disturbing and extremely frightening dreams involving threats to survival, security, or self-esteem. People who have constant nightmares (dream anxiety disorder) may have a genetic basis for this disturbance, but usually there are underlying personality factors and psychological issues. Drugs and alcohol can also affect nightmare frequency and severity.

Q Are there any differences between a child's dreams and an adult's dreams?

Children's dreams differ from adult dreams. Children dream more about animals and family members, and less often about "themselves." Children also have fewer negative emotions in dreams. Studies show that girls have more characters in their dreams, and more domestic situations, than boys. In adolescence, dream content becomes similar to that of adults.

Q Do dreams have any meaning?

Studies show that it is impossible to generalize about individual dreams. This means that the dreams you dream have meaning only for you and are specific to your life. Studies of dream diaries kept by people over many years show that symbols in dreams represent an integration of individual life experiences into the dreams. Some dreams, such as being chased or attacked, are common, but only reflect an emotional state known to us all as anxiety.

Q Where can I find out more about dreams and dreaming?

Sigmund Freud, Carl Jung, and Alfred Adler were the first to bring the unconscious to our attention in modern times, and their works are a good place to start if you're interested in the psychological aspects of dreaming. Bookshops and "new age" shops stock "dream dictionaries," and you can always turn to more scientific studies as well.

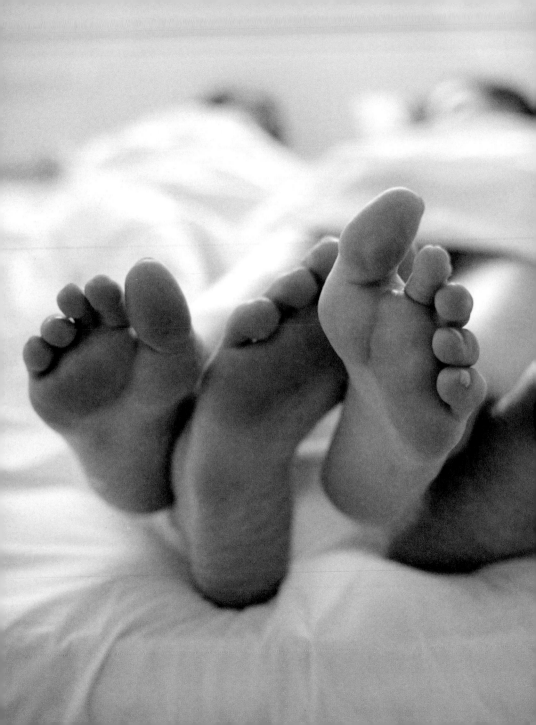

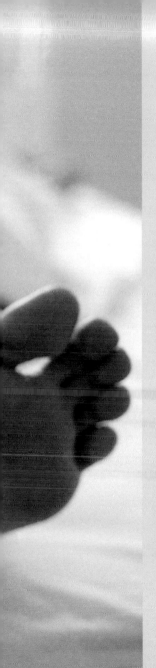

Sleeping well

There are times in our adult lives when we seem to be so overwhelmed by our day-to-day activities that we "forget" what it is like to sleep well, or even how to get to sleep. This chapter focuses on simple strategies to help get you to sleep or improve your sleep and bedtime routines. If you have any concerns at all with any aspects of your sleep routine, it is important to seek professional advice.

Getting enough sleep

Q What is a good night's sleep?

When you wake up feeling refreshed, eager to get out of bed and start the day; when your mind is clear and your mood evenly balanced, you know that you've had a good night's sleep.

Q Is the quality of sleep more important than the quantity of sleep?

Quality and quantity of sleep are equally important in determining a good night's sleep. If sleep is disrupted and not refreshing enough for any reason, the length of time "sleeping" will not improve matters. Similarly, if you do not sleep long enough for your needs, even good quality sleep will not be of much help.

Q Is it important to get to bed at the same time every night?

No. The most important factor determining your bedtime should be your level of sleepiness. If you're not feeling sleepy, getting into bed will just lead you to toss and turn and you will feel frustrated at being unable to get to sleep.

Q Is it important to get out of bed at the same time every morning?

This is much more important than going to bed at the same time every night. Most of us who work get up at the same time every day—we all need to accomplish certain tasks in the morning and get to our workplace or start our work at a certain time. This helps keep the circadian rhythm in check and, therefore, appropriately regulate our levels of sleepiness and wakefulness. An occasional sleep-in won't harm you but generally, if you have a structured week, it is better to keep your sleep-wake schedule regular, even on weekends.

What things are essential for a good night's sleep?

Many factors can help determine whether or not you get a good night's sleep, including the time you go to bed and the time you get up, the environment you sleep in, how much you consume in the way of caffeine, cigarettes, and alcohol (as well as other drugs), and your general well-being. Your mood, lifestyle, and physical health all play a role, as can a number of medical conditions.

IS YOUR LIFESTYLE AFFECTING YOUR SLEEP?

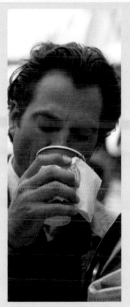

If you think that your lifestyle is leading to sleep disruption, consider the following questions:

- Do you smoke?
- Do you drink more than 6 cups of coffee/tea or 6 glasses or cans of cola a day?
- Do you regularly drink more than 2 units of alcohol (1 pint of beer, 2.5 fluid ounces of sherry, 4.5 fluid ounces of wine or 1.5 fluid ounces of hard liquor would equal 2 units) a day?
- Are you under disruptive stress at home or at work?
- Do you exercise less than twice a week?
- Do you take fewer than 2 weeks' vacation a year?
- Are you dissatisfied, bored, or stuck in a no-win situation?
- Do any of your relationships cause you significant stress?
- Do you generally work more than 10 hours a day or more than 6 days a week?
- Do you never do anything just for the "fun of it"?

Answering "yes" to any of these questions may be an indicator that your lifestyle may be impacting your sleep. If that is the case, it might be time to sit down and reevaluate what is important in your life and how you can minimize stresses and bad habits that can affect both your sleep and your general enjoyment of life.

Myth "You don't need a comfortable bed to get a good night's sleep"

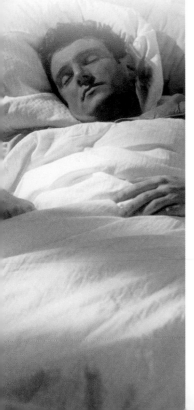

Truth If you're tired enough, you can probably get to sleep anywhere, on a hard floor, in the back of a car on a long journey, or sitting upright in an armchair. However, for sleep that is consistently refreshing you do need a comfortable bed that feels secure. A comfortable mattress in a bedroom that is quiet, dark, and cool, and free of electronic equipment and clutter, is ideal.

Sleeping environments

What is the best environment for sleep?

Most people find that a quiet environment is most conducive to a refreshing sleep, although this can differ on an individual basis. Some people need the absolute quiet of the countryside (no street noise), others feel comforted by "white" noise (noise from fans, air conditioners, or refrigerators), and yet others need a familiar environment with the hum of traffic outside. Generally, less noise is better but it depends on what you are used to.

How important is my bedroom to sleep?

A quiet, cool bedroom provides the best environment for sleeping. If you can afford to, try to use your bedroom only for sleep—don't make it a hub for family activities, your home office, watching TV, or the general living area, especially if you have difficulty sleeping. Sometimes this is not possible but even if your living quarters are tight, it can help if you cordon off the area where you sleep from a certain time at night to when you get up.

Does my bedding or bed influence the way I sleep?

There isn't much in the way of scientific research in this area, but it's commonsense that if your mattress isn't comfortable, your sleep will suffer. Pillows and mattresses don't last forever, so reassess your sleeping environment every so often to make sure your body is getting the support it needs at night. Is there enough room for you (and your partner)? Do you wake up with a stiff neck or a sore back? Mattresses and bedding need to be kept clean, and you should take into consideration how they affect body temperature. A thick woolen blanket in the summer won't help you sleep.

Q How important is the level of light in my bedroom?

Generally, a darker environment is more conducive to sleep. Light affects your circadian rhythm (see p11). Exposure to bright light late at night can potentially postpone your sleep. Likewise, bright light, or the flickering light of a TV, during sleep is disruptive. Some people wake up earlier in summer with the early light and get to bed later. Ways to minimize exposure to bright light include heavy curtains, light-blocking blinds, or an eye-mask. If you live in an area that has very short nights or no darkness in summer (such as Alaska), a room without windows might be the answer.

Q Should I be sleeping in a cool or warm room?

In general, a cool environment is more conducive to sleep because it reflects the fall in the core body temperature during sleep. Although scientists are still debating the temperature that is ideal for sleep, somewhere around 68–77°F (20–25°C) appears to be tolerated by most people and helps sustain sleep. A room that is either too cold or too hot can be uncomfortable and disruptive to sleep. In fact, heat leads to more disrupted REM sleep, increased nocturnal awakenings, and increases in the light stages of NREM sleep.

Q Does humidity make a difference?

Humidity can also be a problem and coupled with heat can make sleep difficult. Air conditioning or a dehumidifier can help with this problem. On the other hand, if the air is too dry, this can lead to discomfort as well. If you are waking up with a sore throat and dry nose (and you're not a snorer or habitual mouth-breather), then this could be due to too little humidity in the air. This can be a problem, especially with heating in winter.

GOOD AND BAD SLEEPING ENVIRONMENTS

Where and how we sleep depends on a myriad of factors, some within and some outside our control. If you have difficulty sleeping, consider some of the factors in your immediate sleeping environment. Sometimes a few small changes can make a large difference. There are no rules about bedroom color schemes or furnishings, as long as they appeal to you.

GOOD ENVIRONMENTS	BAD ENVIRONMENTS
A quiet, cool bedroom that is used predominantly for sleeping (not for work, study, or family activities).	A chaotic bedroom that is cluttered, messy, noisy, and used for too many purposes other than sleep.
A dark bedroom that does not have bright lights and where the curtains block excessive light.	A bedroom that contains a computer, phone, TV, play station, and other digital and electronic devices.
A comforter or blanket that isn't too heavy or too light. Air that is appropriately humidified.	Air that is too dry, uncomfortable bedclothes, or a bedroom temperature that is too hot or cold.
A comfortable mattress, box spring, and pillows that suit your needs.	A worn-out mattress and pillows that are uncomfortable to sleep on.
A welcoming bedroom that is free from clutter and electronic devices.	Pets with a different sleep-wake cycle sharing the bed or bedroom.

Q I find that I am
easily awakened
by noise; what can
I do about it?

As we grow older, our sleep becomes lighter and we are
more prone to disruption of any sort, including noise.
If you find your sleep being disturbed by noise, consider
using the following: ear plugs, sound-proofing measures
such as double-glazing, rugs, roof insulation, "white"
noise to mask other noises (using a fan or a generator),
or relaxing music or tapes. If a noisy or restless co-sleeper
is waking you up with snoring or snoring in association
with breathing pauses, ask him or her to visit a doctor.
In such cases, a separate bedroom also helps, although
this can take its toll on the relationship.

Q Should I have
a clock in
the bedroom?

The bedroom should be a time-free environment.
However, since many people rely on an alarm clock to
wake up in the morning, most of us have a timepiece in
the bedroom. If the ticking of the clock does not disrupt
your sleep or you're not prone to lying awake at night
watching a luminescent digital display screen, then there's
no problem. However, if you are having problems sleeping
and you are a "clock-watcher," then getting the clock out
of the bedroom might improve your sleep.

Q What about pets
in the bedroom?

Again, it is a matter of what you are used to. If you have
always slept in the same room as your pets and don't
find this disturbing, then there is no problem. However,
studies have shown that people who sleep in the same
room as their pets have more nocturnal awakenings and
disruptions than those who don't. Also, if you are allergic
to animal dander your sleep could be worsened. If you
have started having problems with your sleep, then try
sleeping without your pet in the bedroom. It might be a
wrench at first, but eventually it will do you good.

Sleep promotion

Q How do I establish a routine that promotes sleep?

A bedtime routine is part of sleep hygiene and helps you prepare psychologically and physically for sleep. A routine is a way of ordering simple daily tasks and behavioral patterns into a meaningful sequence. If you have difficulty establishing such a routine, it is best to seek help. In addition to assisting you in establishing a routine, a health professional may try a number of different treatments including stimulus control, sleep restriction, and cognitive-behavioral therapy (see p182).

SLEEP HYGIENE HABITS

Try to establish sleep hygiene habits that suit you and your needs. The following tips may help.

- Avoid caffeine, nicotine, and alcohol late in the day.
- Complete the last meal of the day at least 2 hours before bedtime.
- Cut down or avoid fluids at least an hour before bedtime.
- Avoid stimulating environments 2 hours prior to bedtime.
- Engage in exercise but avoid vigorous activity too close to bedtime.
- Use your bed for sleep (and sex) only.
- Don't watch television in bed.
- Establish a bedtime routine.
- Give yourself time to relax before retiring and use relaxation techniques.
- Create a bedroom environment that enhances sleep.
- Think about your concerns and write them down before getting into bed.
- Go to bed only if you are sleepy.
- If you can't get to sleep within 15–20 minutes, get out of bed and do a quiet activity until you're sleepy; repeat if necessary until you're sleepy.
- Get up at the same time every day.
- Avoid daytime naps.

Myth "If you cannot get to sleep, it is best to stay in bed and try harder to sleep"

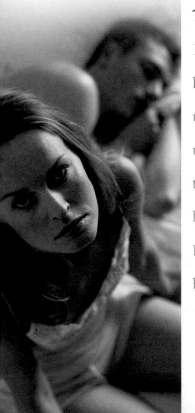

Truth Wrong. If you can't get to sleep within 15–20 minutes, you should get out of bed, leave the bedroom, and do something quiet and unstimulating (like reading a book or knitting) until you feel sleepy again. The longer you toss and turn in bed, the more frustrated and anxious you become and the longer it takes you to get to sleep. If this occurs regularly you'll start associating your bed with sleeplessness rather than sleep.

Q What are the best ways to relax before going to bed?

Relaxation is an important part of preparing for sleep, but there is no best way—you must choose what suits you. There are many forms of relaxation therapy and most are easy for you to do yourself. Progressive muscle relaxation is one useful technique, where you tense and then relax different muscle groups in turn (see p183). Autogenic training also decreases bodily arousal. This involves mental exercises that switch off stress responses and help relax the body's muscles. Some people find listening to soothing music or relaxation tapes helpful. No single relaxation technique has been shown to be more effective than any other.

Q How can I stop my mind racing when I'm trying to go to sleep?

People who are plagued by a continuous stream of thoughts near bedtime can try methods which decrease cognitive arousal, such as imagery training or meditation. Sometimes writing all your worries for the day on a piece of paper and leaving it in a room other than your bedroom can help.

Q Is it all right to nap during the day?

First, ask yourself why you need to have a nap during the day. Are you excessively sleepy, despite spending enough time in bed? Do you have disrupted sleep at night? How often do you nap—after Sunday lunch, once a week, or regularly during the week and at different times? If you do have to have a nap, don't sleep for longer than an hour, because it will affect your level of sleepiness in the evening, and don't nap after 3pm in the afternoon. If you are napping because you find it really hard to keep awake, including at work or while driving, you should discuss this with your doctor.

Q Does regular physical exercise promote a good night's sleep?

In addition to the other health benefits that regular exercise brings to the body, it can also help to improve sleep. Physical exercise tires us out and results in the release of chemicals and hormones in the body that produce better-quality sleep, including the proportion of slow wave sleep that we experience. Exercising in the late afternoon may help you to sleep better; however, vigorous exercise within 3–4 hours of bedtime can interfere with your sleep.

Q Will a bath before bedtime help me to sleep better?

In addition to environmental temperature, variations in our body temperature also play an important role in determining the quality of sleep we have during the night. Our body temperature falls naturally as part of the circadian rhythm toward the end of the day as we prepare to sleep. Having a bath in hot water, at least an hour before going to bed, can help raise the core body temperature and then let it drop more quickly, decreasing the transition time to sleep. Water can also have a relaxing effect on us that also enhances sleepiness.

Q How close to bedtime can I eat?

Regular and scheduled meals throughout the day are important to sustain our energy and provide us with the nutrition our body needs. However, it is best not to go to bed with a full stomach. This disrupts sleep because the body has to work overtime to metabolize the food. A full stomach can also exacerbate heartburn. Conversely, going to bed hungry can also disrupt sleep. Complete your last heavy meal of the day at least 2 hours before going to bed, and if you feel hungry just before retiring, have a light snack.

Q How does drinking water before bedtime affect my sleep?

Many people experience disturbed sleep due to frequent nocturnal urination (nocturia). To minimize this, restrict fluid intake after your last heavy meal of the day, and try not to drink water about an hour before you go to bed. If nocturia persists, seek medical advice.

Q What drugs can help me sleep?

If you have persistent difficulty sleeping (see pp50–81), which leads to impaired daytime performance, it is best to seek medical advice. Drugs prescribed for short-term sleep disturbances include benzodiazepines, such as temazepam, and non-benzodiazepines, such as zolpidem and zopiclone. However, these hypnotics may have side effects and may impair the quality of your sleep. They shouldn't be used for more than 2–4 weeks at a time unless recommended by your doctor. Other drugs that are sometimes prescribed for coping with sleep disturbances and promoting sleep include antidepressants, melatonin, and antihistamines (see pp180–181).

Q What "natural" preparations can help me sleep?

Unfortunately, there is very little scientific data on either the safety or efficacy of herbal preparations and the many over-the-counter insomnia medications that are available. A glass of warm milk (because it contains high amounts of tryptophan, an amino acid) is obviously safe to try, as are the numerous herbal teas that are now commonly marketed. The best medical and scientific evidence available to date for improving sleep and sleep quality in mild insomnia supports the use of valerian or a combination of valerian and hops. See the table on p40 for more information on natural preparations that are potentially conducive to sleep.

SOME NATURAL PREPARATIONS CONSIDERED CONDUCIVE TO SLEEP

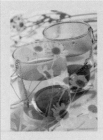

The table lists a number of natural preparations that are often used alone or in combination to aid sleep. If you take conventional medicine for any disorder you *must* tell your doctor you are using herbal preparations because some of them can have dangerous and potentially life-threatening interactions. It is best to obtain herbal teas, pills, or preparations from a licensed herbalist, and many can be purchased in supermarkets and pharmacies.

COMMON NAME	BOTANICAL NAME	FORMULATION
Mint	*Mentha* spp.	Tea; capsules; potpourri
Chamomile	*Matricaria chamomilla*	Tea; potpourri
Lavender	*Lavendula* spp.	Oil; fragrance; tea; potpourri
Hops	*Humulus lupulus*	Capsules; tea mixtures
Lettuce	*Lactuca sativa*	Fresh leaves
Valerian*	*Valeriana officinalis*	Capsules; tea
Purple passionflower	*Passiflora incarnata*	Tea; tea mixtures; pills
Lemon balm	*Melissa officinalis*	Tea; potpourri
Clary sage	*Salvia sclarea*	Tea; tea mixtures
Vervain	*Verbena* spp.	Tea; tea mixtures; potpourri
Oats	*Avena sativa*	Grain; tea

*Do not use valerian if you are taking barbiturates

Q Is it true that tryptophan supplements can help me sleep if I have insomnia?

Possibly, but evidence is limited. Serotonin, a brain chemical that helps promote sleep, is made in the body from the amino acid tryptophan. Low levels of tryptophan have been linked with insomnia. Although supplements are unavailable in the US because of deaths caused by a particular manufacturer, you can try adding foods that contain tryptophan—such as peanuts, almonds, tofu, and meat—to your diet.

Q Can I drink a kava beverage to help me sleep?

Kava (*Piper methysticum*) is definitely not recommended because of its interaction with benzodiazepines. In addition to this, studies of kava were not completed because it showed clear evidence of being toxic to the liver.

Q Can I use melatonin as a "natural" sleeping pill?

There is currently no reliable scientific evidence for the use of melatonin as a sleeping pill. It may be useful in people who have an intrinsic reduction in melatonin production. However, its precise composition, as well as the best way to administer it and the appropriate dose, are still open to debate. Some evidence does exist that it may be useful in the elderly who have nocturnal melatonin deficiency, and may lead to an improvement in sleep efficiency as well as reducing the time it takes to fall asleep (sleep onset time).

Q Are there any vitamin or mineral supplements that help me sleep?

Currently, there is no proven evidence that a particular vitamin preparation will assist with sleep. However, there are a few case reports in which people have responded to vitamin B compounds, especially if they are deficient in these. There is a lack of consistent evidence for the efficacy of calcium, magnesium, copper, iron, or zinc supplements in improving sleep, especially if you are not deficient in these minerals or have a sleep disorder.

Q Do alternative therapies help with sleep problems?

This depends on the type of sleep problem you have. There is anecdotal evidence that therapies such as accupuncture, massage, and homeopathic remedies may be useful in dealing with sleep problems related to lifestyle if they help reduce stress and allow you to focus on yourself. As long as treatment is not harmful, it may be worth trying. However, there are few properly conducted scientific trials to test whether treatments are safe and effective for everyone.

Q How important is it to match sleep patterns with a partner?

If your partner has exactly the same sleep patterns and habits, then you are one of the lucky few. Dealing with differences in sleep patterns always requires some negotiation, compromise, and consideration. If you prefer a cold environment and your partner is a heat-seeker, your partner might have to compromise and consider bedsocks and heavier pajamas. If you are a night owl and your partner an early bird (see p21), you might have to discuss ways of sharing the bedroom to prevent disruption of your sleep patterns. Separate bedrooms can solve extreme differences, but as with many aspects of a relationship, talking openly and constructively about the problem might lead to the solutions that suit you both.

Q Does having sex lead to a better night's sleep?

Very little research has been done to answer this difficult question. For most people, orgasm leads to a release of neurotransmitters, which affect the sleep centers in the brain. However, the effectiveness of sex in inducing sleep depends on how it makes you feel. If it makes you feel peaceful and relaxed, it could help you sleep. If it is a performance, an activity indulged in to prove yourself, or leaves you with high anxiety levels, then it can be the prelude to a night of tossing and turning in bed.

Sleep disrupters

Why can caffeine make sleeping difficult?

Caffeine is a stimulant found in coffee, tea, cocoa, and chocolate, and is an additive in many soft drinks and drugs. It keeps you alert and on the go. Some people are more sensitive to it than others. Caffeine blocks the action of adenosine (see p19) and reduces its sleep-inducing effects in the brain. Caffeine reduces total sleep time and also reduces the amount of slow wave sleep.

How can I cut down on my caffeine intake?

Caffeine enters the bloodstream within 15 minutes of ingestion (for example, drinking a cup of coffee) and shows peak blood levels between 30–60 minutes. To eliminate half the concentration of caffeine in blood takes about 3–5 hours. If you are having difficulty sleeping, cut down on your caffeine intake. Try not to drink any products containing caffeine 4–6 hours before going to bed.

I'm a smoker. What effect does nicotine have on my ability to sleep?

Like caffeine, nicotine is a stimulant. Nicotine withdrawal can occur in heavy smokers once they have gone to bed, and may lead to sleep disruption and nightmares. Generally, it is best to smoke the last cigarette at least half an hour before going to bed to avoid the stimulating effect of nicotine.

What effect does alcohol have on sleep?

Alcohol may make you feel sleepy initially. Larger quantities lead to increased slow wave sleep and suppression of REM sleep early in the night. Later on, a rebound increase in REM sleep can occur as well as more wakenings. This results in unrefreshing sleep. Try to restrict your last alcohol intake to your evening meal.

THE EFFECT OF DRUGS ON SLEEP

Many drugs affect the quality and quantity of sleep we experience, and it is important to be aware of those that are fairly commonly prescribed. Sleeping pills of the benzodiazepine class can suppress slow wave sleep. Many antidepressants can lead to a reduction in REM sleep and some may induce either insomnia or excessive sleepiness. Drug withdrawal can cause a rebound increase in the stage of sleep that was previously suppressed and lead to sleep disturbances. Marijuana in the immediate short term results in minimal sleep disruption with only a slight reduction in REM sleep. Chronic ingestion produces long-term suppression of slow wave sleep. Amphetamines, cocaine, and even drugs used in decongestant mixtures and "sinus relief" tablets, such as pseudoephedrine, can lead to insomnia and significant sleep disturbances.

DRUG	EFFECT ON SLEEP
Alcohol	Suppresses REM sleep; increases frequency of wakenings.
Beta-blockers	Suppress REM sleep; can cause nightmares and increase daytime sleepiness.
Benzodiazepines	Decrease slow wave sleep; can lead to daytime drowsiness, and memory and mood impairment.
Fluoxetine	Affects REM sleep and can cause insomnia.
Phenytoin	Suppresses REM sleep and increases sleepiness.
Pseudoephedrine	Can cause insomnia and sleep disturbances.
Salbutamol	Can cause insomnia; improves sleep if asthma is controlled.
Steroids	Can cause sleep disruption and insomnia.
Simvastatin	Can lead to insomnia.
Theophylline	Increases light sleep; can result in sleep disturbances and insomnia.

Mood and memory

Q Does mood affect the quality of sleep?

Mood can certainly affect your ability to get to sleep or stay asleep. High anxiety levels can lead to a state of hyperarousal (increased alertness), thereby impairing your ability to get to sleep and sometimes to stay asleep. A depressed mood can have varying effects on sleep quality and quantity. Some evidence suggests that, during severe depression, REM sleep starts earlier than normal and may occur more frequently. Severely depressed people spend less time in stage 3 and stage 4 sleep. Some people feel they need to sleep longer, others wake up frequently, and yet others have insomnia, particularly "terminal insomnia" (awakening too early in the morning). If you feel your mood is affecting your sleep patterns, it is best to seek medical advice.

Q What happens to memory as we fall asleep?

Sleep onset closes the gate between short- and long-term memory stores. This means that we don't encode material prior to sleep sufficiently strongly to recall it if sleep persists for approximately 10 minutes. We lose all memory of events that take place a few minutes before sleep onset.

Q Is sleep important for memory?

Yes, many studies have now shown that we need sufficient sleep for our memory to function properly. If we are deprived of sleep our ability to perform well on tasks that require vigilance and concentration, as well as processing of information, markedly decreases. A few studies have shown that even mild to moderate levels of sleep deprivation can produce a level of functioning similar to being drunk.

Sleep diary

How do you know you are sleeping consistently well? One way of monitoring your sleep and sleep patterns is to keep a sleep diary. Like all diaries, it helps to record your activities during the day and particularly the amount of time you spend asleep. Sometimes we are unaware of our bad habits until they are pointed out to us. The diary helps you uncover any factors leading to poor sleep. It is also a way of monitoring change or progress and in particular, the treatments or changes in your behavior that may help you sleep better.

Keep your sleep diary beside your bed and fill it in every morning for 2 weeks— you can use the example opposite for reference. Indicate for each day any events that may have influenced or disturbed your sleep. If you do have concerns about the quality of your sleep or sleep patterns, seek medical advice.

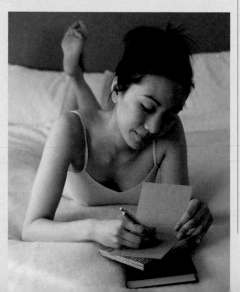

ACTIVITIES (ABBREVIATIONS)

A = each alcoholic drink

C = each caffeinated drink (such as coffee, tea, cola, chocolate)

P = every time you take a sleeping pill or tranquilizer

M = meals

S = snacks

X = exercise

T = use of toilet during sleep time

N = noise that disturbs your sleep

W = time of wake-up alarm, if any

SLEEP TIME

Shade in box for every hour you were asleep

Hatch in box for every hour you were lying down, unable to sleep

EXAMPLE SLEEP DIARY – WEEK 1													
	MON		**TUE**		**WED**		**THUR**		**FRI**		**SAT**		**SUN**	
	A	**ST**	**A**	**ST**	**A**	**ST**	**A**	**ST**	**A**	**ST**	**A**	**ST**	**A**	**ST**
6am														
7am	W		W		W				W					
8am	C/S		C/S		C/S		W		C/S		N		T	
9am							C/S							
10am					C				C		W/M			
11am	C		C				C				S			
12 noon													C	
1pm	M		M/A		A		M		M			H	M/A	
2pm					M				C					
3pm			C								C/M		X	
4pm	C/S						C						X/S	
5pm														
6pm	A		C		C				A		C			
7pm	X				X		M		A					
8pm	M		M		M				M/A				M	
9pm	C		C		A						M/A		C	
10pm					A/S				A					
11pm									A/S					
12 midnight			N											
1am														
2am	T													
3am									T					
4am					T									
5am														
TST (hrs)		8		6½		6½		7½		5		7½		7½

A = activities

ST = sleep time (including naps)   Total sleep time (TST) .... hrs

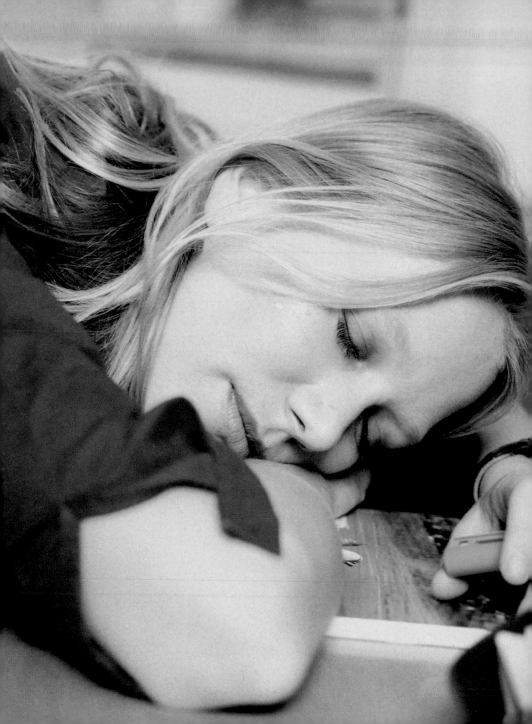

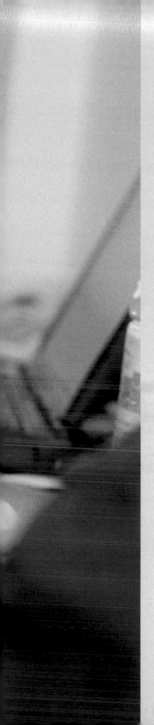

Sleep disorders

Disorders relating to sleep
contribute to impaired academic
and job performance. They
can result in accidents and can
also affect mood and social
adjustment. Relationships can
be severely affected by the
disordered sleep of a bed partner.
Sleep disorders can lead to or
worsen underlying medical and
psychiatric problems. The good
news is that most sleep disorders
can be treated.

Disrupted sleep

Q **What is a sleep disorder?**

A sleep disorder is an abnormality in the state or progression of sleep. It disrupts sleep and can manifest itself in symptoms, such as daytime sleepiness.

Q **What are the different kinds of sleep disorders?**

Sleep disorders are either primary, when they are intrinsic to the sleep process, or secondary, when the sleep disruption or abnormality results from another disease in the mind or body. Primary sleep disorders encompass the following: disorders that cause insomnia, disorders of excessive daytime sleepiness, sleep-disordered breathing (abnormal breathing rhythms in sleep), disorders of excessive movement during sleep, disorders in the timing of sleep (as in jet lag), and disorders resulting in abnormal events during the night, such as sleepwalking.

Q **What are the symptoms of a sleep disorder?**

The most common symptoms are inability to get to sleep or maintain sleep (insomnia), excessive daytime sleepiness, nocturnal awakenings, or abnormal movement, behavior, or sensations during sleep.

Q **What is daytime sleepiness?**

This is a feeling of not being alert or as alert as one should be during the day. It is important to distinguish between sleepiness and physical fatigue, and to be clear in your mind how you really feel.

Q **How do I know if I am excessively sleepy?**

You will know this yourself. For a more objective assessment, medical professionals use various tools to gauge the level of subjective and objective sleepiness. One such tool is the Epworth Sleepiness Scale (see p51).

THE EPWORTH SLEEPINESS SCALE

The Epworth Sleepiness Scale was first devised by Dr. Murray Johns in Australia and published in 1991. It measures chronic sleepiness over time. It has been extensively validated and translated into many languages, and is one of the most widely used clinical questionnaires in the world today.

This scale asks how likely are you to doze off or fall asleep in a number of situations, in contrast to feeling just tired. It refers to your usual way of life in recent times. Even if you haven't been in some of these situations recently, try to work out how they would have affected you. Use the following scale to choose the most appropriate number for each situation:

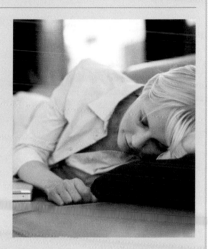

(0) = no chance of dozing

(1) = slight chance of dozing

(2) = moderate chance of dozing

(3) = high chance of dozing

SITUATION	CHANCE OF DOZING
• Sitting and reading	(0) (1) (2) (3)
• Watching television	(0) (1) (2) (3)
• Sitting inactive in a public place (like a theatre or a meeting)	(0) (1) (2) (3)
• As a passenger in a car for an hour without a break	(0) (1) (2) (3)
• Lying down to rest in the afternoon when circumstances permit	(0) (1) (2) (3)
• Sitting and talking to someone	(0) (1) (2) (3)
• Sitting quietly after a lunch without alcohol	(0) (1) (2) (3)
• In a car, while stopped for a few minutes in traffic	(0) (1) (2) (3)

Add up your score, which could be a maximum of 24. A score of 11 and over is consistent with excessive daytime sleepiness.

Myth "Sleep disorders are neither common, nor serious"

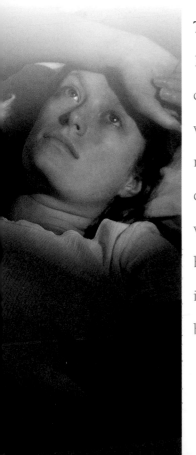

Truth At any one time, approximately 10 percent of the population suffers from a clinically significant sleep disorder. In other words, 1 in 10 people have a condition that requires a doctor's advice or treatment. Sleep disorders can result in accidents at work and while driving, thereby raising significant public health issues. The most common sleep disorder is insomnia, followed by sleep-disordered breathing, and restless legs syndrome.

Insomnia

What is insomnia?

Insomnia is the term used to describe inadequate or poor-quality sleep that may be due to one or more of the following: difficulty falling asleep, difficulty staying asleep, waking up too early in the morning and being unable to get back to sleep, and unrefreshing sleep.

How does insomnia affect daytime functioning?

Insomnia results in unrefreshing sleep and can lead to daytime problems of fatigue, lack of energy, difficulty concentrating, and irritability.

Are there different types of insomnia?

Periods of sleep difficulty lasting between one night and a few weeks are referred to as acute (transient) insomnia. Chronic insomnia refers to sleep difficulty during at least 3 nights a week for 1 month or more.

How common is insomnia?

Insomnia is the most common complaint that is related to sleep and wakefulness. About 30–40 adults out of 100 have some degree of insomnia within any given year and about 10–15 in 100 indicate that the insomnia is chronic or severe. Insomnia increases with age and is more common in women. Women are about 1.3 times more likely to report insomnia-like sleep problems than men are. People over 65 years of age generally have approximately 1.5 times higher rates of difficulty sleeping compared with adults below the age of 65. Children can also have problems with insomnia and the rates for adolescents are similar to adults. Sleep onset insomnia is most common in young people.

Q What causes insomnia?

Insomnia is nearly always related to a medical, psychiatric, circadian, sleep, behavioral, lifestyle, or environmental disorder. Acute insomnia is closely related to a major life event, such as pregnancy, significant stress at work, or bereavement. Once the event loses its intensity, the insomnia should also lessen. The development of chronic insomnia is often complex. An important factor appears to be a tendency to hyperarousal, or increased alertness during the day and night. People with hyperarousal have increased anxiety, and a higher heart rate while sleeping.

Q What are the consequences of insomnia?

Insomnia can result in excessive sleepiness during the day, which can impact on activities such as driving and the operation of machinery, as well as decrease in concentration and ability to learn. Other consequences can relate to mood. Many people with ongoing insomnia become depressed or generally agitated. Insomnia can also worsen an underlying medical condition.

Q How is insomnia treated?

Acute insomnia can be treated with short-term use of sedative medications such as benzodiazepines. Good sleep hygiene is mandatory (see pp35), and some herbal preparations (see pp40) may be useful. People with chronic insomnia must combine treatments such as relaxation techniques (see p183), using the bedroom only for sleeping, setting regular sleep patterns, environmental change, treatment of medical/mood problems, and the judicious use of medication. People with chronic insomnia may benefit from counseling or cognitive-behavioral therapy (see p182). Not all treatments apply to or are effective in every individual with insomnia. If you have insomnia, discuss your treatment with your doctor.

Narcolepsy and abnormal daytime sleepiness

Q What is narcolepsy?

Narcolepsy was first described in 1880. It is characterized by an abnormal need to sleep, often in inappropriate situations. Nocturnal sleep is often disturbed.

Q What are the symptoms of narcolepsy?

The main symptoms are excessive daytime sleepiness, attacks of muscle weakness called cataplexy, sleep paralysis (transient inability to move as you fall asleep or wake up), and visual hallucinations (see p56).

Q How common is narcolepsy?

Classic narcolepsy is rare but it has many variations that are more common. Some 20–50 people in 100,000 have the condition. Between 1 and 4 in 10 people with narcolepsy have a family member who is also affected. Rarely, narcolepsy can be passed on through the genes. It can be a major social disability. Almost all patients with narcolepsy have a special genetic marker in the blood which can be tested for. Narcolepsy is now known to be due to a deficiency of the substance hypocretin (orexin) in the brain and spinal cord. Very rarely, the symptoms of narcolepsy may appear following a brain injury or in association with diseases of the central nervous system.

Q At what age does narcolepsy start?

Narcolepsy usually appears between the ages of 15 and 30; sometimes it can start before the age of 10, or may not be recognized until after 50 years of age or even older. It is a lifelong condition.

Q How is narcolepsy diagnosed?

Narcolepsy can be confirmed by doing an overnight sleep study followed by a special test called the multiple sleep latency test (MSLT). This test involves having 4–5 separate naps over the course of the day, assessing the time it takes for a person to get to sleep, and also whether dreaming sleep occurs. A special blood test is used to look at the genetic make up of the person to support a diagnosis of narcolepsy. A diagnosis of narcolepsy is made on the basis of the symptoms that the patient reports and the results of more objective testing as mentioned above.

THE SYMPTOMS OF NARCOLEPSY

Excessive daytime sleepiness. People with narcolepsy can have anywhere from 2 to 30 episodes of uncontrollably falling asleep during the day. These attacks can occur at any time, even if a person is working. Each sleep attack can be as short as a few seconds and up to 20 minutes in duration. Following a sleep attack, they feel refreshed.

Cataplexy. Cataplexy is muscular weakness caused by strong emotions such as laughter. Cataplexy attacks commonly occur in situations involving perfectly normal emotions, such as humor (hearing or telling a joke), competitiveness (bidding in a game of bridge), excitement (viewing, or especially participating in, a sports event), and stress or self-assertion.

Sleep paralysis. This is a short period of inability to move during sleep, and it can last from a few seconds to half an hour. It is due to loss of postural muscle tone.

Hypnagogic hallucinations. A hypnagogic hallucination is best described as visual hallucinations or dreamlike images ("awake dreaming") that can occur at the start of sleep.

Is narcolepsy a severe condition?

If mild, the symptoms of narcolepsy may cause no more than minor inconveniences. If severe, however, symptoms can cause significant disruptions in one's social and professional life, and may become profoundly disabling. Parents, teachers, spouses, and employers may often mistake sleepiness for lack of interest, or as a sign of hostility, rejection, or laziness.

How is narcolepsy treated?

The sleepiness associated with narcolepsy can generally be greatly improved by the regular use of stimulant medication, such as modafinil (see p181). At present, these stimulant medications are the only drugs available. For cataplexy, antidepressant medication (such as clomipramine and imipramine) can be very helpful. The drug sodium oxybate can also be useful in instances of severe cataplexy.

Can narcoleptics drive a vehicle?

If symptoms are well under control, narcoleptics can continue driving under normal conditions, and if they are being seen by a doctor at least once a year to discuss their symptoms and their medication. It is the responsibility of the person with narcolepsy to notify their insurance company and the appropriate licensing authority of their condition.

What are the other disorders of excessive daytime sleepiness?

A few other disorders can make you sleep a lot during the day, like idiopathic hypersomnolence (idiopathic means "without a cause," hypersomnolence means "excessive sleepiness"). Most are rare and the diagnosis can only be made by a sleep specialist or physician. Some people who sleep in excess are naturally "long sleepers" but this diagnosis is made only if all other disorders are excluded.

Sleep-disordered breathing

Q **What are the types of sleep-disordered breathing?**

There are several types, the most common is snoring, followed by sleep apnea caused by upper airway obstruction. Another type is central sleep apnea, which may occur in people with severe heart failure, but can also occur spontaneously or in association with neurological conditions such as strokes. Obesity hypoventilation syndrome is another type of sleep-disordered breathing in which the morbidly obese person can have significant breathing pauses during the night, leading to respiratory failure.

Q **What is sleep apnea?**

Sleep apnea is a form of sleep-disordered breathing where there are breathing pauses—air entry into the lungs is temporary halted—despite continued effort to take a breath. Sleep apnea is said to occur when the pauses last for 10 or more seconds and are repeated regularly throughout the night. The common symptoms are snoring and choking that may lead to awakening during the night. Very often, the person with sleep apnea is unaware of the problem and of being sleepy during the day, and it is the bed partner who brings it to medical attention.

Q **How common is sleep apnea?**

Sleep apnea is very common, affecting more than 4 of 100 people in the middle-aged population, and is more common than either diabetes or asthma. The chances of developing sleep-disordered breathing become more common with increasing weight and age but it can affect anyone at any age, from babies to the elderly.

What are the daytime symptoms of sleep apnea?

Over 9 in 10 people with sleep apnea experience excessive daytime somnolence, or abnormal sleepiness. This can lead to driving impairment, intellectual impairment, personality changes, mood disturbances, reduced libido/impotence, marital disharmony, irritability, and a reduced quality of life.

What are the night-time signs of possible sleep apnea?

These signs are usually reported to the person with sleep apnea by a bed partner; occasionally the person is aware of the events themselves. Snoring is the most common event and occurs in 90–95 percent of all cases. Other signs include witnessed breathing pauses (75 percent), a dry mouth in the morning (75 percent), excessive sweating (50 percent), choking attacks (25 percent), and urination at night (25 percent). An absence of snoring does NOT exclude sleep apnea.

What causes the breathing pauses in sleep apnea?

In sleep, the muscle tone of the upper airway (pharynx) tends to narrow and collapses temporarily. This results in repetitive breathing pauses accompanied by a drop in blood oxygen levels and arousal from sleep, and leads to daytime symptoms of sleep apnea.

What are the risk factors for the development of sleep apnea?

Being male, middle-aged, and obese (see p60) confers the greatest risk of developing sleep apnea. Other risk factors include mild abnormalities of the jaw and facial structure, such as an overbite or a smaller lower jaw. The structure of the face, especially the middle, and the shape of the hard palate, nasal blockage, and problems with breathing through the nose, as well as large tonsils, adenoids, and a large tongue, can all lead to sleep apnea. Between 30 and 50 percent of people with sleep apnea are NOT obese.

Calculating body mass index (BMI)

People who are obese are at greater risk of developing sleep apnea than people who are a healthy weight for their height. People with a BMI of 30 or more are usually considered obese. BMI can be precisely calculated by dividing your weight in pounds by the square of your height in inches and multiplying the result by 703. However, for women, adding to 100 pounds, 5 pounds for every inch over 5 feet tall for women, or, for men, adding to 106 pounds, 6 pounds for every inch over 5 feet tall will put you in the center of your ideal weight.

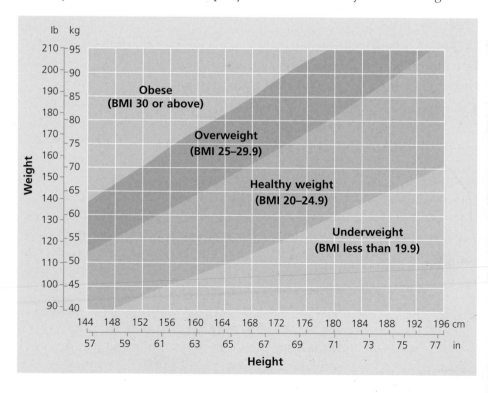

Is the type of obesity important in the development of sleep apnea?

Central obesity with a high waist:hip ratio is a greater risk for the development of sleep apnoea. That means that people with an apple-shaped body (excess weight around the waist) are generally at greater risk than people with a pear-shaped body (weight around the hips). See p60 to find out how to determine if you are overweight.

What makes sleep apnea worse?

Alcohol can worsen sleep apnea by reducing the activity of the upper airway and dilating muscles that prevent the airway from closing over during sleep. Sedatives have a similar effect; they also have the potential of reducing respiratory drive. Sleep deprivation, nasal congestion, and sleeping on your back can also worsen sleep apnea.

Does sleep apnea have any other effects on health?

Sleep apnea may contribute directly to conditions such as high blood pressure (hypertension) and there is a possible association with heart attacks and strokes. Severe sleep apnea can lead to increased breathing risks while being anesthetized for surgery. Sleep apnea can lead to problems with concentration and memory, and is associated with depression and mood impairment.

How is sleep apnea diagnosed?

Sleep apnea syndrome is diagnosed on the basis of symptoms of excessive daytime sleepiness and an overnight sleep study to objectively document breathing pauses. This can be done using a variety of methods, including full PSG (polysomnography) or home-based sleep studies with more limited apparatus. It could simply involve a probe on the finger (oximeter) to look at overnight breathing patterns and the changing levels of oxygen in the blood (oxygen saturation patterns). An experienced sleep technologist will score and assist in the interpretation of the study data.

Treating sleep apnea with CPAP

Continuous positive airway pressure (CPAP) is currently considered the "gold standard" treatment for moderate to severe obstructive sleep apnea. There is a large variety of machines, all of which are designed to generate an airstream that keeps the upper airway open during sleep. The choice of machine and the level of air pressure will be determined by a sleep specialist, usually after the patient undergoes an overnight study at a sleep center.

FACE MASK OPTIONS

People who use continuous positive airway pressure may take a little time to adjust to using their mask, but a range of different styles and designs are available and most users are able to find one that fits well and is comfortable to wear.

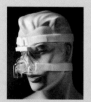

NASAL MASK   FULL FACE MASK

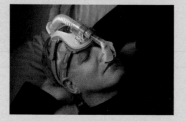

NASAL PILLOW

Nasal masks, the most common type, sit over the nose, where they are held in place with a strap around the head.

Full face masks are particularly useful for patients who only breathe through their mouth or whose breathing alternates regularly between their nose and their mouth.

Nasal cushions or pillows are inserted into the nostrils. They offer a useful alternative to nasal masks for people who experience claustrophobia from masks or for people who cannot get an ideal mask fit.

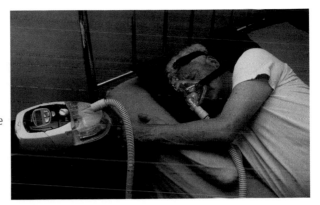

A GOOD NIGHT'S SLEEP
The supply of a steady airstream from a CPAP device splints the airway open, prevents breathing pauses and gives the user a good night's sleep.

ALTERNATIVES TO FIXED CPAP

Occasionally, patients may find it uncomfortable to breathe out against a fixed pressure or CPAP may be difficult to tolerate. They may benefit from devices designed to provide a variable pressure that automatically adjusts to their breathing at night or from bi-level positive pressure ventilation using a different type of machine.

AUTOTITRATING CPAP DEVICES

Sometimes known as "intelligent" CPAP, these devices use a pressure sensor (or occasionally a flow oscillation technique) to analyze air flow and adapt the pressure to the patient's needs over the course of the night. This enables the device to deliver the lowest pressure necessary to maintain an open airway, thereby making it more comfortable to use. Autotitrating CPAP devices tend to be more expensive than fixed pressure machines, but prices may decrease with time.

BI-LEVEL POSITIVE PRESSURE

This ia a form of ventilation frequently used in patients who have respiratory failure (see p88), with or without obstructive sleep apnea. Occasionally, it is used if CPAP alone cannot be tolerated due to the extremely high pressures required to keep the airway open at night. Bi-level positive pressure systems deliver a higher pressure on inhaling (breathing in) and a lower pressure on exhaling (breathing out). See also p89 for treatment of respiratory failure.

Q How is sleep apnea treated?

The best treatment for moderate to severe sleep apnea is using a machine that generates continuous positive airway pressure (see pp62–63). Milder forms of sleep apnea can be treated using a mouth-guard splint, called a mandibular repositioning splint, which is constructed by a prosthodontist, orthodontist, or dentist. The device acts by pulling the lower jaw forward and opening the airspace at the back of the throat.

Q Are there lifestyle measures that will help?

Weight loss (if you are overweight or obese) can help reduce the severity of sleep apnea. Cut out alcohol, particularly before bedtime, don't take sedatives, and if you smoke, quit. Not sleeping on your back may help if your apnea occurs only in that position, and can be achieved with positional training.

Q Is surgery an option for treating sleep apnea?

Surgery is usually not recommended for moderate to severe apnea but there are circumstances when it may be useful. For example, if the tonsils or adenoids are too large, they can be removed. If the soft palate and uvula are too big they can be reduced with laser-assisted uvulopalatoplasty (LAUP) or supported with a palatal strut, both of which are brief, outpatient procedures. Jaw deformities can also be corrected.

Q Can people with sleep apnea drive?

The risk of a motor vehicle accident is increased seven-fold in the presence of sleep apnea (all other risks being equal). Once sleep apnea is adequately treated and the person is no longer abnormally sleepy, then driving should not be a problem. A person with sleep apnea should notify his or her insurance company and the Department of Motor Vehicles.

Snoring

What is snoring?

Snoring is defined as a type of breathing during sleep accompanied by harsh or hoarse sounds caused by the vibration of the soft palate and other tissues at the back of the throat. Breathing occurs through the open mouth and nose. Snoring is a subjective experience on the part of the person forced to listen to it.

Is snoring the same as sleep apnea?

No. Snoring occurs in 90 percent or more of people with sleep apnea but is not the same condition. Snoring is the sound made by vibration of the soft palate without episodes of apnea (breathing pauses) or hypoventilation (shallow breathing).

What are some of the potential consequences of snoring?

Very loud and persistent snoring commonly leads to severe strains on relationships because of the sleep disruption it causes. Snoring can lead to multiple arousals (wakefulness during the night) and severe sleep fragmentation. Both of these disturbances can result in excessive sleepiness during the day.

What can I do about my snoring?

Lifestyle factors contribute to snoring and modification of these can sometimes lessen the degree and intensity with which you snore. These include losing weight (if you are overweight or obese), not sleeping on your back, avoiding alcohol before bedtime, quitting smoking, and treating nasal congestion. It is important that your doctor also excludes any anatomical abnormalities that can contribute to snoring or worsen it, including adenoids, large tonsils, jaw problems, and nasal blockages.

Myth "Snoring is just a nuisance and it is best to joke about it"

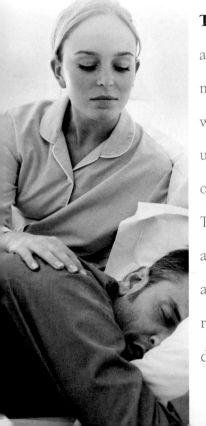

Truth Snoring is far from being just a nuisance and is rarely a joke either for those who snore or, more importantly, for people who have to put up with their snoring. Persistent snoring can put an unbearable strain on relationships, even neighborly ones, and can lead to various medical problems. There is some evidence that people who snore have an increased risk of developing high blood pressure and that women who snore may have higher-risk pregnancies with detrimental effects on the developing fetus.

Are there any good devices that may help my partner stop snoring?

Mandibular repositioning splints (MRS) are probably the best devices we have currently for treating snoring—especially if it's simple—and mild sleep apnea. These oral appliances are shaped like gum shields or mouthguards, and are worn over the teeth at night during sleep. The idea is to hold the lower jaw forward, thereby opening the airspace at the back of the throat. In some instances, they are called mandibular advancement devices (MAD). Mandibular repositioning splints should be made by a dentist, orthodontist, or prosthodontist. Good evidence exists to show that they work if constructed properly by an experienced professional.

Are there any other devices that might help?

Adhesive external nasal dilator strips (ENDS) are often suggested as a way of preventing snoring. However, large trials have not revealed any convincing evidence that they cause significant improvement in snoring. Mouthguards bought over the counter are generally useless. If a partner is disturbed by snoring, ear plugs or sleeping in another room can help in extreme cases of very disruptive snoring. CPAP (pp62–63) can be useful.

Is surgery useful in treating snoring?

If there is no evidence of sleep apnea after an overnight sleep study or problems with sleepiness during the day because of snoring, then surgery *may* be useful. If you are considering a surgical solution to your snoring, you must see a specialist for an assessment. There are a number of different techniques used to treat snoring surgically, but overall the success rates are low, ranging from 20–50 percent maximum 6 years after the surgery. Remember that some techniques have never been subjected to proper clinical trials, so be very careful.

Limb movement disorders

Q What are limb movement disorders?

These are disorders of excessive movement during the night that are not explained by any other abnormality or medical condition. They include periodic limb movement disorder and restless legs syndrome (RLS), which is quite common.

Q What are the symptoms of RLS?

The symptoms of RLS include unpleasant feelings in the limbs, especially in the calf muscles. They can occur in both legs and can also occasionally affect the arms. People with RLS usually report unpleasant sensations that they describe as being crawling, tingling, burning, and aching. These symptoms are made worse by rest and are helped by activity of the affected limb, although they often recur a few minutes after activity has ceased. People with RLS are unable to remain still, particularly in the evening or at night, and often have difficulty sleeping.

Q How is RLS diagnosed?

Frequently, if a sleep study is performed, people who are suspected of having RLS are found to have repetitive regular leg movements that can disturb their sleep and leave them tired during the daytime. Often, however, the person is able to provide an accurate medical history that confirms the diagnosis of RLS.

Q When does RLS occur?

RLS typically occurs at the end of the day when you relax or get into bed. It may also occur during the day if you are in a confining spot, such as a theater, plane seat, or on a long car ride.

How common is RLS?

RLS affects more than 5 in 100 adults. In many people, it can start before the age of 20 years. However, RLS is more common with increasing age. Several large family studies have suggested that it tends to run in families. It can occur during pregnancy but usually ceases after delivery of the baby. RLS is present in about 50 percent of people with kidney failure on dialysis. It can also occur if there are low iron stores in the blood or a deficiency of folate (folic acid). RLS can be associated with other neurological conditions, such as Parkinson's disease (see p118–119). It can also occur in rheumatoid arthritis or if the thyroid gland is underactive. Some antidepressant medications can cause RLS, and it has also been reported in people with varicose veins in their legs.

How is RLS treated?

RLS may be difficult to treat but usually responds well to medication and some general measures. The latter include relaxation techniques (see p183), massage of the limbs, and avoiding all stimulants, such as coffee, tea, cola, and over-the-counter decongestants. There are many medications that can be used in the treatment of RLS. However, not all of them work for every individual and might be effective for varying periods of time. Some of the more commonly used medications for RLS include: sedating medications such as the benzodiazepines, anti-Parkinsonian agents, analgesic (pain-killing) medications, and anticonvulsant drugs. Iron supplements may also help. Sometimes, medications become less effective with time and must be changed.

Disorders in the timing of sleep

Q What types of disorders affect timing of sleep?

There are a number of problems that can affect the timing of sleep. These disorders generally involve either voluntary or involuntary disruption of the body's circadian rhythm (see p11). The most common are shift-work disorder, jet lag, and delayed sleep phase syndrome (see p76).

Q What is jet lag?

Our body clock adjusts very slowly in response to abrupt changes in environmental time cues. No change is probably more abrupt than that of air travel across several time zones. Jet lag is characterized by a group of symptoms, such as inappropriate daytime fatigue, insomnia, early waking, disturbed sleep patterns, and impaired concentration and alertness during the day. Other symptoms include loss of appetite, inappropriate toilet times, and excessive urination at night.

Q Is jet lag worse traveling eastward or traveling westward?

Traveling eastward shortens the day to less than 24 hours and traveling westward does the opposite. It is easier to postpone falling asleep than trying to get to sleep earlier than usual (which happens when we travel east). Traveling westward generally leads to quicker adaptation to local times. However, the severity of symptoms also depends on other factors, including the number of time zones crossed, flight duration, and your circadian system's adaptibility to changes. About a third of people who fly do not experience any significant effects of jet lag.

Is melatonin useful in combating jet lag?

There is some evidence that melatonin, if taken appropriately, may assist with decreasing the symptoms of jet lag, largely by helping the body adjust to a different sleep-wake schedule. The usual dose that has been tested in studies is 5mg (see below for timing of doses, depending on whether you are traveling east or west). Melatonin can reduce alertness and induce sleepiness so you MUST NOT drive or operate heavy or dangerous machinery once you have taken it. Short-term use of melatonin appears to be safe although very little of the available data supports this claim. The most common side effects are sleepiness, headache, and nausea. The long-term effects on health are currently unknown, although there is some evidence that there are detrimental side effects (see p18). Always use a licensed, quality-controlled melatonin preparation.

If I travel EAST over several time zones, when should I take melatonin?

On the day of departure, take a dose of melatonin between 6 and 7pm local time (place of departure). On arrival at your destination, take melatonin at the local bedtime (10–11pm) for 4 days. If your stopover is shorter than 4 days, on the evening preceding your departure back home, do not take a capsule at bedtime but at 6–7pm local time. On arrival, take melatonin daily for 4 days at your usual bedtime if you need to.

If I travel WEST over several time zones, when should I take melatonin?

Do not take any melatonin before the flight. When you reach your destination, take a dose of melatonin at the local bedtime (10–11pm) or later, for 4 days. If you wake up very early in the morning (say around 4am) you can take another dose, but be aware that this can make you feel very sleepy the next day.

Reducing the effects of jet lag

When you travel by air across several time zones (see below), your sleep-wake cycle and the levels of melatonin in your body are initially out of kilter with the local day-night cycle at your destination. This can lead to the various symptoms of jet lag (see p70). To reduce the effects of jet lag, try to follow the advice on the opposite page, which will help you synchronize your body clock to local conditions. Avoiding natural bright light at the wrong time is probably the most important factor in reducing jet lag.

TRAVELING THROUGH TIME ZONES

The world is divided into 24 zones of local time, which correspond to every 15 degrees of longitude and the 24 hours of a day. However, as a result of political and regional issues the time-zone map of the world does not consist of equally spaced lines (see below).

Whether you fly from east to west or from west to east, the more time zones you cross the more jet lag you are liable to experience. Many people report that their jet lag is worse when they fly from west to east, which is the same direction in which the Earth spins on its axis.

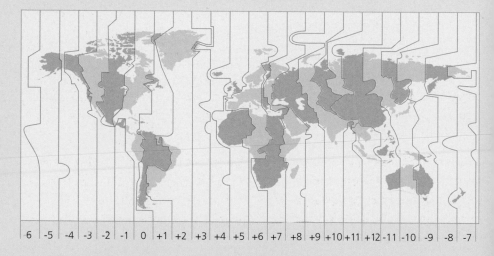

| -6 | -5 | -4 | -3 | -2 | -1 | 0 | +1 | +2 | +3 | +4 | +5 | +6 | +7 | +8 | +9 | +10 | +11 | +12 | -11 | -10 | -9 | -8 | -7 |

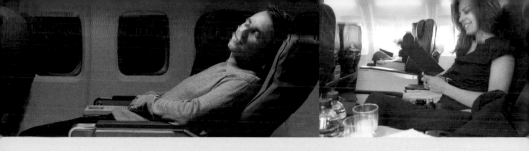

ADVICE FOR REDUCING JET LAG

Before you go Use a calculator to help you figure out the best way to time your exposure to light before and after your trip. Several calculators can be accessed for free on the Internet—for example, www.bodyclock.com.

Rest Try to be as well rested as possible before you travel. Getting on the flight exhausted or stressed will not improve your trip.

Comfort If you can afford it, fly business or first class so you can rest adequately during the flight (especially if you're flying for business reasons). If you are traveling in economy class, try to ensure that you have as much room around your seat as possible (minimize the bulk of your hand luggage). Get up and stretch your legs on a regular basis.

Sleep If you are traveling on a night flight, try to get some sleep. Recline your seat and use the eye shades to shut out the cabin light and ear plugs to minimize the noise.

Food, drink, and exercise Drink plenty of water during the flight, stretch regularly, and walk around in the plane if possible. Avoid alcohol and caffeinated drinks, such as tea, coffee, and colas, because they cause water loss and can disrupt your rest. Eat light meals.

Once you arrive On arrival at your destination, try to fit your sleep–wake pattern to the pattern at your destination. For instance, if you arrive early in the morning, expose yourself to daylight and try to stay awake. If you arrive in the evening, try to go to bed at a reasonable bedtime for you.

Medication Hypnotic medications that are short-acting can be useful to ensure that you sleep not only during the flight, but also on arrival at your destination.

Melatonin There is some evidence that, if properly timed, melatonin can assist with alleviating jet lag (see p71). Always use a licensed, quality-controlled preparation of melatonin.

Q What is meant by shift-work disorder?

Sleep problems and other health problems arising from working schedules outside normal daylight hours can result in shift-work disorder. This disorder results from the interaction of social and domestic, circadian rhythm, and sleep factors.

Q Who is prone to shift-work disorder?

Although some people cope well with irregular working shifts, those who are most likely to develop problems include people over the age of 50, those with a history of sleep disorders (like sleep apnea or narcolepsy), those with diabetes, epilepsy, heart disease, digestive problems, psychiatric problems, or a history of alcohol or drug abuse. Other factors that can impair tolerance to shift-work include a heavy domestic workload, more than one job, and being a morning person (an "early bird").

Q Can the type of shift you work lead to shift-work disorder?

Drawing up an appropriate shift-work roster is crucial for optimizing performance and minimizing problems in coping with shifts. Shifts that are harmful to well-being include: 12-hour shifts involving monitoring tasks, heavy physical labor or exposure to harmful substances, more than four 12-hour night shifts in a row, very early morning shifts, split shifts with inadequate breaks, weekly rotations, and more than 5 late-night shifts in a row.

Q What is the impact on health of long-term shift-work?

People who work shifts have an increased risk of heart disease, breast cancer, and high blood pressure, and many also have digestive tract problems. Disrupted time with the family can have significant impacts on people's lives. Permanent shift-workers often have an increased risk of mood disorders, especially depression, and abuse of alcohol and drugs. Sleep is never entirely normal.

What can I do to minimize the negative impact of shift-work on my life?

As well as the tips in the box below, sedatives or stimulants can be useful to regulate the sleep-wake pattern but must be prescribed by a doctor. Weigh up the pros and cons of shift-work and how you adapt to it. "Night owls" tend to do better than "early birds." After middle age, shift-work becomes more difficult due to changes in our sleep patterns with ageing. If you have a medical condition, reconsider whether shift-work is right for you. Changing jobs or negotiating for alternate shifts may be an answer.

STRATEGIES FOR DEALING WITH SHIFT-WORK

Here are some tips you can follow for you to sleep better if you are a shift-worker:

- Optimize your sleep hygiene (see p35). Eye shades and ear plugs are especially useful if you sleep during the day.
- Attention to bedroom environment. Try to keep the bedroom cool, dark, and as quiet as possible.
- Exercise regularly. Avoid strenuous exercise before bedtime.
- Plan to end your sleep as close to the start of the shift as possible. If necessary, take a nap before the night shift.
- Eat a balanced diet. Smaller meals are better for those starting a night shift.
- Avoid caffeine and bright light before the end of a night shift

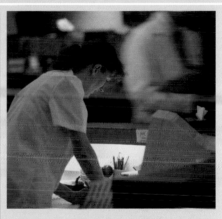

to prevent delays in getting to sleep. In very bright environments, wear sunglasses when you are traveling home.
- If you are very sleepy at the end of the night shift, make safe travel arrangements to get home or take a nap before setting off.

Q What is delayed sleep phase syndrome (DSPS)?

This is a circadian rhythm disorder with an exaggerated "night owl" pattern of sleep and wakefulness. Generally, speaking, a person with delayed sleep phase syndrome (DSPS) has sleep onset and waking times that are delayed by 3–6 hours compared to conventional sleep-wake times. A person with DSPS feels sleepy and is ready to go to bed at about 2–6am and gets up by 10am–1pm. Sleep itself is normal. This sleep-wake pattern must be present for at least 3 consecutive months for diagnosis of the condition.

Q How common is DSPS?

DSPS can occur from childhood into old age. It is more common in adolescents and young adults. Estimates suggest that about 7 in 100 adolescents and young adults have DSPS.

Q What are the symptoms of DSPS?

People with DSPS cannot get to sleep before early morning and have difficulty getting up in the morning at appropriate times. They may complain of daytime fatigue and this may lead to impairment of school and job performance. They are most tired in the morning and increasingly feel more alert during the day.

Q What causes DSPS?

A combination of factors results in DSPS. There are genetic factors associated with the genes regulating the circadian rhythm—some cases of DSPS definitely run in families. There may be subtle problems in the regulation of the circadian rhythm (see p11) and also with the ability to recover normal sleep patterns. Behavior and lifestyle factors that involve continued disruption of the circadian rhythms plays a strong role in reinforcing DSPS.

How is DSPS diagnosed?

A sleep specialist can diagnose DSPS by using techniques such as actigraphy (see p178) and polysomnography if necessary (see pp14, 176). In addition, sleep diaries (see pp46–47) and the general history of the complaint can both contribute to the diagnosis.

How is DSPS treated?

A number of different methods may be used to treat the timing problem involved in DSPS and resetting the sleep-wake pattern. These include light therapy in the morning or skipping one night of sleep and "resetting" bedtime at the desired hour the next night. This should be done under the supervision of a sleep specialist. The person may take melatonin before bedtime.

What is advanced sleep phase syndrome (ASPS)?

This disorder of the circadian rhythm is the opposite of DSPS. Sleep is normal but a person has a sleep-wake schedule about 3 hours earlier than average. A person with ASPS is very sleepy in the late afternoon and early evening, and goes to bed early in the evening. They get up early—anywhere between 2am to 5am. The causes, diagnosis, and treatment of ASPS are similar to those of DSPS but targeted at different times of the day and phases of the circadian rhythm. About 1 percent of middle-aged adults have ASPS but it is generally not considered a socially incapacitating problem. People with ASPS often gravitate toward jobs that suit their extreme early morning habits.

What other circadian rhythm disorders are there?

Other disorders include non-24 hour rhythms, in which the sleep-wake cycle does not run on the rhythm of a normal 24-hour day. Certain forms of blindness can cause problems with circadian rhythms and timing of sleep.

Parasomnias

Q What are parasomnias?

Parasomnias are disorders resulting in abnormal events during the night, such as sleep-walking, night terrors, bruxism (tooth-grinding), nocturnal groaning, enuresis (bedwetting), rhythmic rocking movement disorder, and sleep-talking. Most can be divided into disorders that affect either REM or NREM sleep. Some parasomnias are not confined to any particular sleep stage.

Q What can trigger an abnormal event during sleep?

A number of factors can trigger a parasomnia or make it occur more frequently. These factors include fever, alcohol, prior sleep deprivation, strenuous physical activity, emotional stress, and various medications. Parasomnias can also be made worse by pregnancy or menstruation, and sleep-disordered breathing (see p58). Genetic and environmental factors often interact to cause parasomnias.

Q When should medical help be sought with a parasomnia?

Bizarre, sleep-related activities may occasionally be experienced by normal people and usually do not warrant further investigation or treatment. However, you may need to seek medical advice if the affected person's behavior is violent/injurious, disruptive, results in excessive daytime sleepiness, or is associated with medical, psychiatric, or neurological symptoms and findings.

Q How is a parasomnia diagnosed?

A history of the person's unusual behavior is noted. It is helpful if family members can recount behavior they've witnessed. The disorder may be investigated further with the person spending a night in a sleep center and undergoing PSG (see p14) with video recording.

Normal and abnormal events during sleep

Some events that occur during both NREM and REM sleep are considered normal, while other events are thought to be abnormal (see below). Medical advice should always be sought if you are unsure about the symptoms you are experiencing. It is helpful if someone in your household can also describe the behavior that you are experiencing. If the behavior is disruptive to you or to others, it should be investigated.

NORMAL EVENTS DURING NREM AND REM SLEEP

NREM sleep	REM sleep
• Sleep starts (see p17)	• Sleep paralysis (see p56)
• Sensation of the head exploding	• Hallucinations while falling asleep and waking up; usually occur only when sleep-deprived

ABNORMAL EVENTS DURING NREM AND REM SLEEP

NREM sleep	REM sleep
• Sexual behavior during sleep	• REM sleep behavior disorder (see pp80–81)
• Confusional arousals (waking up confused and distressed)	• REM-related painful erections
• Sleep-walking (see pp80–81)	• Dream anxiety attacks (nightmares)
• Sleep terrors (see pp80–81)	

Q What is sleep-walking?

Sleep-walking consists of a series of complex behaviors that are initiated in NREM slow wave sleep and result in walking during sleep. It is also called somnambulism or noctambulism. Sleep-walking may terminate spontaneously or the sleep-walker may return to bed, oblivious to the fact that they left it in the first place. Occasionally, there is also inappropriate behavior. Falls and injuries may occur if the person walks into dangerous situations, like out of a door and into the street or through a window. Rarely, aggressive behavior occurs, especially as a response to attempts to restrict the sleep-walker's mobility; homicide or suicide have also been reported. Contrary to popular belief, it is not dangerous to wake a sleep-walker.

Q How common is sleep-walking?

Sleep-walking occurs regularly in 1–3 in 100 children, and occurs occasionally in about 1 in 4. It usually disappears after adolescence. Sleep-walking occurs regularly in 1–6 in 1,000 adults and occasionally in 1–3 in 100. Sleep-walking is hereditary and about 85 in 100 adults who do sleep-walk have had the condition since childhood.

Q What are night terrors?

Also known as *pavor nocturnus* (in children) or *incubus* (in adults), night terrors are characterized by a sudden arousal from NREM slow wave sleep with a piercing scream or cry, accompanied by manifestations of intense fear. The attacks usually end spontaneously. Night terrors occur regularly in 3 in 100 children and occasionally in about 10 in 100 children. They usually end during adolescence and less than 1 in 100 adults experience them.

What is sleep-talking?

Sleep-talking is the utterance of speech or sounds during sleep without the person being aware of the event. No one knows why people talk in their sleep, although there may be a link with an anxiety disorder or a fever. Sleep-talking is usually brief, infrequent, and devoid of signs of emotional stress. Some sleep-talkers seem to be able to hold conversations, while most just moan, say the odd word, or make unintelligible sounds. Sleep-talking occurs regularly in 4–14 in 100 children, and occasionally in more than 1 in 4. Sleep-talking occurs regularly in 1 in 20 adults, and occasionally in about 1 in 3.

Is there any treatment for sleep-talking, sleep-walking, and night terrors?

Treatment should be discussed with a medical expert. If the behaviors occur infrequently, then no specific treatment is usually necessary. If the behaviors are causing problems, then several medications can be used to treat them. Occasionally, psychotherapy, progressive relaxation and hypnosis can be useful.

What is REM-behavior disorder?

This is a disorder that can occur at any age, but is more common in middle-aged to older men. It occurs during REM sleep when a person tries to act out their dreams, usually in a violent or disturbing manner. Instead of the body being paralyzed, as is normal in REM sleep, it is able to act out the dream. People with REM-behavior disorder can often injure themselves and their partners, sometimes seriously. REM-behavior disorder can occur spontaneously, as part of another sleep disorder, such as narcolepsy, or as the first sign of other neurological disorders, such as Parkinson's disease (see pp118–119). The disorder can be treated but should always be diagnosed and managed by a sleep specialist.

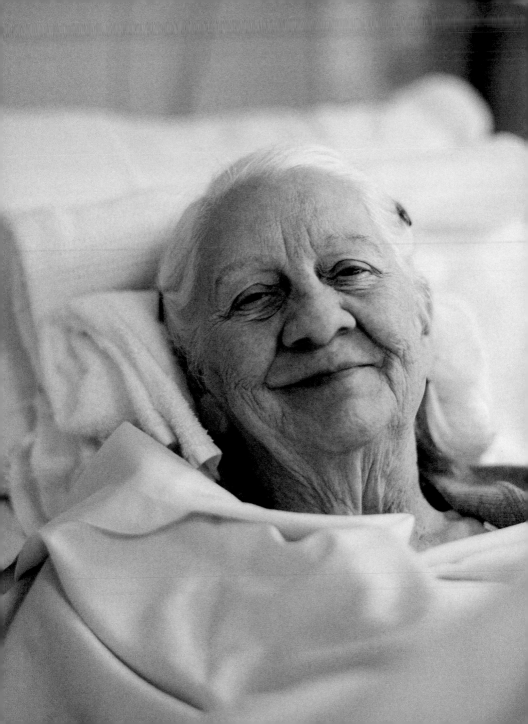

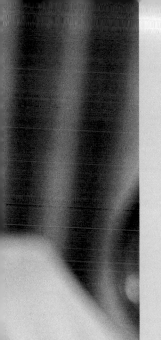

Illness, aging, and sleep

Sleep is essential to the maintenance of health. Any disease process that impacts on our well-being will affect our sleep. This chapter deals with sleep in the context of illness, disordered mood, and pain. Also discussed are sleep in aging and the effect of medication on sleep. We have all experienced the restorative powers of a good night's sleep when sick, and the corollary is also true— poor-quality sleep slows recovery and impacts negatively on our well-being.

Respiratory disorders

Q **What are the common respiratory disorders most likely to affect sleep?**

Respiratory disorders affect the breathing passages and lungs, muscles of breathing, breathing centers in the brain, and the space around the lungs (pleural space). Any respiratory illness that affects breathing can disrupt sleep. The most common respiratory conditions in the US are asthma and chronic obstructive pulmonary disease (COPD). People with respiratory failure (breathing difficulties due to muscle weakness, lung disease, or severe obesity) can also have increased problems with breathing at night.

Q **Can asthma affect sleep quality?**

Over two-thirds of people with asthma experience narrowing of their airways during the night. This explains why the symptoms of many asthmatics worsen at night or early in the morning as evidenced by cough, wheeze, or breathlessness.

Q **Why does airway narrowing (broncho-constriction) occur at night?**

There is no single reason. In normal people, there are circadian changes in bronchoconstriction with a decrease in airway caliber at night. This response is exaggerated in asthmatics. Other factors that can cause airway narrowing include sleeping position, allergens in bedding, reflux, and impairment of mucous transport in the airways at night.

Q **How does nocturnal wheeze affect sleep?**

Sleep is disrupted by the mechanics of coughing and the inability to get enough air into the lungs. This causes the oxygen level in the blood to fall. If the disruption is significant enough, it will lead to symptoms of daytime sleepiness. Although death from asthma is rare, most deaths from asthma occur at night or early morning.

What can I do about my nocturnal asthma symptoms?

Nocturnal bronchoconstriction is a definite sign of poor asthma control and you should seek medical advice about your asthma condition. Long-acting beta2-agonist inhalers are useful and the addition of a steroid inhaler may be necessary to reduce airway inflammation leading to bronchoconstriction. If you also suffer from sleep apnea, treatment of this condition will also improve asthma control. People with gastroesophageal reflux also benefit from acid suppression therapies. Keeping a regular peak flow meter chart will allow you to assess your progress and help your doctor work out a medication regimen for you.

I have been diagnosed with COPD. How could this affect my sleep?

If your COPD (chronic obstructive pulmonary disease) is moderate to severe, you could experience periods of low blood oxygen levels during the night. Generally, your oxygen levels will fall at first during REM sleep and then as the disease progresses, during NREM as well. Low oxygen at night may make you feel unrefreshed in the morning and contribute to more restless sleep.

What causes oxygen levels to fall during the night in COPD?

You will probably already be experiencing lower oxygen levels during the day due to destruction of lung tissue responsible for transferring oxygen from the lungs into the blood. During the night, as muscles relax, oxygen levels drop further because you are breathing less during sleep. This is the most likely explanation for low oxygen levels at night in people with moderate to severe COPD. Once oxygen levels start to deteriorate, carbon dioxide levels build up and can lead to morning headaches and feelings of nausea as well as fatigue and sleepiness during the day. If someone has concurrent sleep apnea, then the problem can be worsened significantly.

Myth "Disease does not affect either the quality or quantity of sleep"

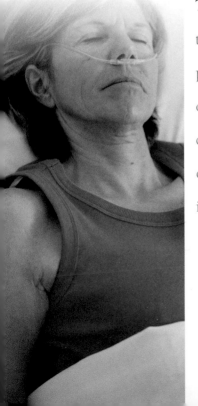

Truth This is not true. It is important to recognize that even in the absence of a primary sleep disorder, such as sleep apnea or narcolepsy, sleep and daytime functioning can be significantly affected by other medical or mood disorders as well as by pain, whether it be short-term or chronic.

How does low oxygen affect the body?

Long-term low oxygen levels in the body can lead to heart rhythm problems as well as problems with increasing pressure on the right side of the heart, leading to heart failure with fluid buildup in the body. Sometimes, overproduction of hemoglobin to high levels occurs to deal with the low oxygen levels in the body, and this can also lead to problems.

Should I have a sleep study to find out what my oxygen levels are during the night?

If your oxygen saturation as measured by the doctor is less than about 85 percent during the day while breathing room air at rest, your oxygen levels are probably dropping during the night, thereby leading to unrefreshing sleep. Overnight monitoring of your oxygen saturation using a probe on the finger (oximeter) is the first step toward being assessed.

What happens if my oxygen levels are low?

If your oxygen saturations drop significantly during the night as determined by your doctor, you may benefit from overnight oxygen delivered by nasal prongs to your nose. However, oxygen therapy is prescribed only to people who do not smoke. If you have carbon dioxide retention during the day as well as low oxygen, which your doctor can determine by doing a blood gas test, then you may benefit from other forms of treatment, with or without additional oxygen therapy. At that stage, you should be referred to a respiratory or sleep specialist who will assess you further.

Can I use sedatives for my insomnia if I have COPD?

This depends on how severe your COPD is and how low your oxygen levels are. All sedatives must be used with caution: your doctor will be able to discuss the possible options with you.

WHAT IS CHRONIC RESPIRATORY FAILURE?

Chronic respiratory failure is of 2 types: in Type 1, not enough oxygen enters the bloodstream from the lungs but the carbon dioxide levels stay low; in Type 2, oxygen levels are low and carbon dioxide levels high. In someone with normal breathing, oxygen levels are high and carbon dioxide levels are low. The types of conditions in which people develop respiratory failure are outlined below:

AREA OF BODY	CONDITIONS ASSOCIATED WITH RESPIRATORY FAILURE
Lungs and airways	• Pulmonary fibrosis (scarring of the lung tissue) • Pulmonary vascular disease (disease of the arteries and veins of the lungs) • COPD (chronic obstructive pulmonary disease) • Bronchiectasis (abnormally wide airways with excessive mucus production) • Cystic fibrosis
Rib cage	• Kyphoscoliosis (excessive curvature of the spine) • Thoracoplasty (deforming surgery to the ribcage) • Obesity hypoventilation (diminished drive to breathe due to massive obesity)
Central nervous system	• Central alveolar hypoventilation (diminished or absent drive to breathe)
Muscles and nerves	• Cervical cord lesions (injuries to the spinal cord in the neck) • Motor neuron disease (progressive degeneration of the nerves in the brain and spinal cord that control muscles) • Poliomyelitis • Post-polio syndrome (muscle weakness and fatigue many years after recovering from polio) • Muscular dystrophies and myopathies (muscle disorders resulting in muscle weakness)

What happens during sleep in respiratory failure?

In the early stages, gas exchange is relatively well preserved in NREM sleep; it is only during REM sleep when our body is "paralyzed" that breathing might not be adequate to compensate for breathing difficulties. Oxygen levels can dip sharply and carbon dioxide levels rise. As breathing problems grow more severe, the drop in oxygen and rise in carbon dioxide starts to occur throughout all stages of sleep and will then persist during the daytime. This leads to the symptoms of moderate to severe Type 2 respiratory failure.

What are the symptoms of Type 2 respiratory failure?

Type 2 respiratory failure can give rise to a number of symptoms including shortness of breath; poor sleep quality with nightmares, insomnia, and arousals; early morning headaches; fatigue, sleepiness, and loss of energy; reduced daytime performance; loss of appetite and weight loss.

How is respiratory failure treated?

Your doctor will advise you on this. You should be referred to a lung or sleep specialist who will examine you, do tests, and assess your breathing. Some people benefit from a treatment called noninvasive ventilation (see below).

How does noninvasive ventilation work?

As you inhale, a machine delivers room air under pressure into your airway. This augments your own breathing and allows the muscles of ventilation to rest. When successful, central control of breathing improves. The pressure is delivered through a mask, similar to that used in continuous positive airway pressure (CPAP; see p62). Oxygen may be added to increase overnight oxygen levels.

Can I use sedatives if I have respiratory failure?

It depends on how severe your respiratory failure is and how low your oxygen levels are. All sedatives must be used with caution, so discuss this with your doctor.

Hormonal imbalances, heart disease, and indigestion

Q What are the common hormonal imbalances?

Hormones play an important role in the regulation of metabolism, growth, and sexual function. Abnormalities in the level of hormones such as insulin and thyroid hormone can affect many systems and organs in the body. Most hormonal imbalances are rare, with diabetes mellitus and thyroid disease being the most common in the US. In fact, these are so common that they should be tested for if anyone complains of fatigue during the day.

Q How do inadequate amounts of thyroid hormone affect sleep?

Low levels of thyroid hormone (hypothyroidism) can cause a drop in the amount of slow wave sleep. The most important sleep link with hypothyroidism is sleep apnea (see pp58–64), which does not go away if just your hypothyroidism is treated—so it is important to be treated for both conditions.

Q How does diabetes affect sleep?

No specific abnormalities in sleep have been noted with diabetes. Obviously, having a hypoglycemic attack during sleep can be dangerous because it can be missed and may make you lethargic in the morning. Many people with sleep apnea have diabetes or are in a prediabetic stage. Sleep apnea is often under-recognized in the diabetic population. If you have diabetes and think you may have symptoms of sleep apnea, it is important that you consult your doctor.

How does hyperthyroidism (high levels of thyroid hormone) affect sleep?

If you produce too much thyroid hormone, your metabolism increases greatly and not surprisingly, can lead to problems with insomnia. This may result in daytime mood changes and exacerbate your already low frustration and tolerance levels as well as increase your irritability. Treatment of hyperthyroidism will settle this down and help restore more restful sleep. During this phase of the illness, sedative medication may be helpful.

What is the link between heart disease and sleep?

A large number of heart conditions can be affected by normal hormonal and nervous system changes that occur during sleep. Studies in large populations suggest that about 1 in 5 heart attacks and about 1 in 6 sudden cardiac deaths occur in the hours between midnight and 6am. This nocturnal risk of worsening heart disease may be a result of the fact that many people are unaware of their symptoms while they are asleep at night.

How can sleep increase the risk of having a heart attack?

During the different stages of sleep, there are changes in hormonal levels and the action of the nervous system in the body responsible for "fight or flight" responses (the sympathetic and parasympathetic systems). Sleep-induced instability in these systems can cause increased strain on an already sick heart and lead to problems with heart rhythm and rate, angina, and heart attacks. Some cardiac medications and medications taken for high blood pressure can also trigger violent dreams (thereby increasing activity) and cause poor sleep. Having a sleep disorder such as sleep apnea also increases the risk of heart strain.

Q What can I do to ensure that my sleep is not putting my heart at any risk?

Firstly, all people with heart disease should examine their lifestyle and make sure that they are at their ideal weight, exercising within their limitations, taking their medications, eating well, not smoking or drinking alcohol excessively, and having regular checkups with their cardiologist. Those who think that their medications are causing problems, or that they may have sleep apnea (which is a major risk factor for heart attack), should discuss it with their doctor. Effective blood pressure control and reporting any heart-related symptoms that occur at night are crucial to managing the condition.

Q How does heart failure affect sleep?

Heart failure, if it is poorly controlled or very severe, can cause nocturnal waking, often with a sensation of shortness of breath and panic. Sleep apnea can coexist with heart failure and also disrupt sleep. Sometimes people with severe heart failure can experience breathing pauses because of poor circulation to the respiratory control centers in the brain. This can add to feelings of daytime fatigue and sleepiness. None of the experiences described above are "normal," so if you have any of these symptoms you must talk to your doctor. A specialist should investigate breathing disruptions in heart failure so that you are treated appropriately for the condition.

Q What digestive problems can affect sleep?

Any problems with the digestive system can disrupt sleep during the night and lead to a feeling of being unrefreshed during the day. The most common problems are uncontrolled diarrhea resulting from an infection of the gut, inflammatory bowel disease that is poorly controlled, or irritable bowel disease. Problems with acid reflux (heartburn) are also very common.

I have problems with heartburn (acid reflux) at night —is this normal?

About 7 in 100 otherwise "healthy" people experience heartburn on an almost daily basis. Most of these people also experience significant heartburn at night, disrupting sleep and leading to feeling unrefreshed in the morning. Many of us will experience occasional heartburn, often after spicy food, or if a large meal is eaten close to bedtime. Nocturnal reflux may be a sign of sleep apnea.

What can I do about my heartburn at night?

There are simple lifestyle measures you can take to reduce the degree of heartburn. These involve eating smaller meals in the evening, several hours before going to bed. Elevation of the head of the bed can also be useful (you can buy a special bed or use bricks to prop up the head of the bed and create a tilt). Sometimes, people find it useful to use several pillows so that they are not lying completely flat. An antacid may also be useful. Avoiding foods that provoke your heartburn is a good idea and avoiding alcohol before bedtime is also recommended. However, if your heartburn persists, you must seek medical advice. Investigation and treatment are now fairly straightforward. Untreated heartburn increases the risk of peptic ulcers and, in the long term, of developing esophageal cancer.

Why is heartburn worse at night?

There are many factors that can contribute to worsening of heartburn at night, including the position that we sleep in and a reduction in swallowing frequency and salivation (production of saliva) during sleep. Thus, acid that refluxes up the esophagus tends not to be washed back down into the stomach. Acid secretion in the stomach is also enhanced during the night. Alcohol and sedative medication can delay acid clearance, making reflux worse.

Sleep and cancer

Q What causes fatigue in cancer patients?

Various factors can contribute to fatigue in people suffering from cancer. Physical factors include weight loss and increased catabolism (tissue breakdown), problems with bone marrow function (leading to anemia, for example), abnormalities in hormone secretion, and salt and fluid imbalances. Psychological problems like depression and anxiety can lead to fatigue. Sleep—and circadian rhythm—disruption can also lead to fatigue and feelings of sleepiness. Treatments such as chemotherapy and radiation therapy can cause significant fatigue.

Q What is the difference between fatigue and sleepiness?

Since there is no single treatment for fatigue in cancer, it is important to know the difference between these two descriptions for problems that can impair quality of life so much. Fatigue is a term that describes feelings of muscle weakness and lack of energy, but without sleepiness. Sleepiness is associated with a desire to fall asleep or unintended episodes of falling asleep in the daytime.

Q How is sleepiness treated in cancer?

Sleepiness in cancer can be due to many factors, including a primary sleep disorder existing before the cancer was diagnosed. If, for instance, someone with cancer has sleep apnea, then the latter should be treated just as in anyone without cancer. If a cancer drug or chemotherapy has led to a sleep-related movement disorder (e.g. restless legs), that disorder should be treated specifically. If depression has developed, therapy should treat the mood disorder. In addition to drug treatments, general sleep hygiene measures should be followed (see p35).

How is fatigue treated in cancer?

Your doctor must try to determine whether there is a specific cause for the fatigue. This includes making sure that your body's biochemical balance is in order, that any anemia is corrected, any infection is treated, and any hormonal imbalance is brought under control. Some of these disorders can develop as a result of cancer treatment with various drugs. Nausea, vomiting, and pain need to be treated as well. Physical activity often reduces the sensation of fatigue. Mild exercise, such as a walk outdoors, can increase light exposure, help fight depression, and train sleep-wake times. Cancer pain must be controlled too. Drugs are also available to combat daytime fatigue.

Can better timing of cancer treatments help treat fatigue?

There is some new evidence to suggest that timing cancer treatments to coincide with circadian rhythms of the body can help decrease the feelings of fatigue, improve quality of life, and lead to less nausea. If chemotherapy is timed to coincide with the rhythms of the body, then sometimes even higher doses of medication can be used with fewer side effects. Research in this area is continuing.

Can drugs used in the treatment of cancer pain cause sleepiness?

Many different types of drugs are used in the treatment of cancer pain, ranging from acetaminophen through nonsteroidal anti-inflammatory drugs (NSAIDs), to morphine and its derivatives. Morphine can certainly induce drowsiness, so if you are feeling sleepier than you would like to be, then you must discuss the dose you are receiving with your doctor. Sedative medication, such as the benzodiazepines, is commonly used for the treatment of insomnia in cancer and can lead to a "hangover" effect the next day. If you have any concerns, you must discuss these with your doctor.

Sleep and pain

Q What is pain?

Pain, as defined by the International Association for the Study of Pain, is an "unpleasant sensory and emotional experience associated with actual or potential tissue damage or described in terms of such damage."

Q What is acute pain?

Acute pain is pain that is typically short-lasting, where relief is readily available and, if properly treated, it may not result in a long-term negative impact on quality of life or health. An example of acute pain is a toothache or wound pain after an operation.

Q What is chronic pain?

Chronic pain is longer lasting. If pain lasts weeks to months and cannot be controlled, it can result in poor quality of life and impairment of day-to-day activities, work performance, and relationships. If the emotional and mood aspects of chronic pain are not appropriately managed, severe problems can result as well.

Q How does pain disrupt sleep?

Pain that occurs acutely (such as wound pain immediately after surgery, angina, or a severe toothache) can disrupt sleep by delaying sleep onset, causing awakening from sleep or poor sleep quality. However, this type of pain is usually short-term and once treated, the effects on sleep are immediately reversible. Chronic pain, even if low-grade and long-lasting, can lead to a vicious cycle (see p97) where sleep is disrupted leading to poor sleep and increased pain sensitivity the next day. This cycle then continues and affects mood, energy, behavior, and one's general safety during the day.

How common is poor sleep in chronic pain?

It is estimated that up to 1 in 4 adults experience chronic pain, and that more than half of these people experience sleep disturbances irrespective of what is causing the pain.

What other types of sleep disruption, apart from insomnia, occur in chronic pain?

Apart from insomnia, chronic pain sufferers can experience nightmares, periodic limb movements, sleep apnea, sweating, and heart palpitations. Patients on high levels of morphine or related analgesics can have breathing pauses at the start of sleep related to instability of the respiratory centers in the brain.

THE VICIOUS CYCLE OF PAIN

Acute pain can lead to poor sleep in the short term, but this is reversible as long as the individual returns to having good sleep or manages the pain so that sleep is unaffected. If the pain becomes chronic, however, and affects sleep in the longer term, it can lead to a vicious cycle: lack of sleep makes the pain more intense and this in turn disturbs sleep.

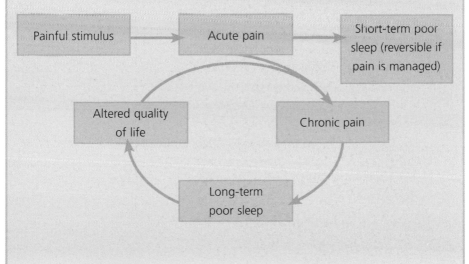

Q **What causes sleep disruption in chronic pain?**

Chronic pain results in sleep fragmentation and arousals leading to poor quality, unrefreshing sleep. Sleep fragmentation can result in an absolute increase in stage 1 and stage 2 sleep in relation to the other stages of sleep. This means that there is less slow wave sleep which is considered restorative to physical processes. People with chronic pain also experience many microawakenings during the night related to body movement. There also appears to be overactivation of the sympathetic nervous system in people with chronic pain, which leads to increased anxiety, and problems with maintaining and initiating sleep, leading to insomnia.

Q **What are the daytime symptoms in chronic pain?**

Poorly controlled pain and poor sleep can lead to fatigue, excessive sleepiness during the day, headaches, sleepiness while driving, anxiety, anger, and frustration.

Q **How are sleep problems in chronic pain treated?**

Control of pain and any associated mood disorder is the key to treating sleep disturbances in chronic pain. Your doctor should use an incremental and multipronged approach. This includes determining whether you might have a primary sleep disorder (see pp50–81) and reviewing sleep hygiene issues with you (see p35). Your doctor will also work out whether talking therapies, such as cognitive-behavioral therapy (see p182), or physical therapies, such as massage or TENS, might be useful. Your doctor may then try medication, nerve blocks, and other ways to control pain. There are many medications that can be used for both treating pain and inducing sleep and these must be tested under medical supervision. Treatment of chronic pain is complex and referral to a chronic pain specialist or clinic is advisable.

Sleep and mood disorders

How does depression affect sleep?

Depression can cause sleep disturbances ranging from insomnia or disturbing dreams to too much sleep time. Several factors are involved in disturbed sleep including increased levels of anxiety and arousal, abnormalities in circadian rhythm (some of which may be affected by drugs used in treating mood disorders), and the fact that the brain and neurochemical systems involved in regulating the sleep-wake cycle are also involved in mood regulation. Both sleep disturbance and fatigue have the greatest predictive value for the presence of a depressive illness. Sleep studies on patients with depression show problems with sleep continuity, decreased slow wave sleep, and abnormalities in REM sleep, among other findings.

How are sleep disturbances treated in people with mood disorders?

If a major depression is present, you need to see a doctor or psychiatrist. There are many different and effective medications for treating depression. Not all people will respond to the same medication and you might have to try several different medications to find the ideal one. Most drugs for depression function by altering the brain's neurochemical balances. Many take several weeks to work and treatment should continue for at least 6 months.

What other forms of treatment are there for depression?

Cognitive-behavioral and other talking therapies may be useful adjuncts to treatment of depression depending on its severity. Sleep deprivation and light therapy can be used as alternatives or in conjunction with medication, even if the depression is nonseasonal. However, these treatments must only be undertaken with appropriate medical guidance.

Could I be depressed?

The following questions are based on a questionnaire known as the Zung self-rated depression scale, and can be used to assess the presence and severity of mild degrees of mood disorder. They can be used from adolescence onward. The questions are not a substitute for a professional diagnosis, so if you are at all concerned about your symptoms, then it is best to seek medical advice—you can fill the questionnaire out and take it to your doctor for further assessment.

Read each statement below and place a tick in the column that applies to you. Each question relates to how you have felt in the last week. Don't take too long thinking about your answer

Make check mark in appropriate column	A little of the time	Some of the time	Most of the time	All of the time
I feel down-hearted and blue	①	②	③	④
I feel best in the morning	④	③	②	①
I have crying spells or feel like crying	①	②	③	④
I have problems sleeping at night	①	②	③	④
I still eat as much as I used to	④	③	②	①
I still enjoy sex	④	③	②	①
I notice that I am losing weight	①	②	③	④
I have trouble with constipation	①	②	③	④
My heart beats faster than usual	①	②	③	④
I feel tired for no reason	①	②	③	④

because the questionnaire is designed to assess your mood and will be more accurate this way. Add up the number of points you score. The maximum score is 80. Scores above 50 are suggestive of depression. If you scored above 50, or are concerned that you may be depressed, you must discuss this with a health professional.

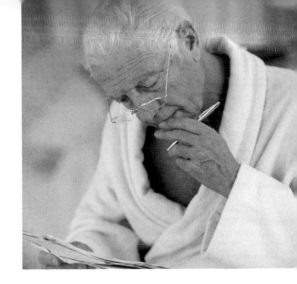

Make check mark in appropriate column	A little of the time	Some of the time	Most of the time	All of the time
My mind is as clear as it used to be	④	③	②	①
It is easy to do the things I used to do	④	③	②	①
I feel restless and can't keep still	①	②	③	④
I feel hopeful about the future	④	③	②	①
I feel more irritable than usual	①	②	③	④
I find it easy to make decisions	④	③	②	①
I feel that I am useful and needed	④	③	②	①
I feel my life is pretty full	④	③	②	①
I enjoy the things I used to do	④	③	②	①
I feel that others would be better off if I were dead	①	②	③	④

Q How does schizophrenia affect sleep?

Schizophrenia is a devastating neuropsychiatric illness with a prevalence worldwide of about 1 in 100. The precise cause of schizophrenia is unknown. The impact on sleep of this illness is variable. Patients with psychotic agitation can have long periods of sleeplessness. Insomnia is the most common problem in schizophrenia and is often characterized by a reduced total sleep time, sleep fragmented by periods of wakefulness, and problems getting to sleep. Some patients experience a reversal of their sleep-wake patterns, preferring to stay awake all night and sleep during the daytime. Some patients experience nightmares and also a greater frequency of hypnagogic hallucinations (the visual hallucinations or dreamlike images that can occur at the start of sleep). Substance and alcohol abuse can worsen these problems.

Q How do anxiety disorders impact on sleep?

One manifestation of an anxiety disorder is the presence of panic attacks. These can occur during sleep and are characterized by an intense feeling of fear and anxiety accompanied by palpitations, chest pain, light-headedness, and nausea (among other symptoms). The presence of nocturnal panic attacks can lead to a worsening of the anxiety disorder and to all sorts of maladjustments with respect to sleep hygiene and sleep. Many people with anxiety disorders also experience depression and the major sleep problem is insomnia. Anxiety disorders can be made worse by lifestyle habits, such as excessive caffeine intake or smoking, so sleep hygiene measures can help with sleep. Other treatments include medication and talking therapies, which often prove to be very effective.

How is sleep affected in bipolar disorder?

During the manic episode there is a decreased need for sleep, which is generally not perceived to be a problem by the patient. During a depressive phase, sleep disturbances are just like those described for depression (see p99). Difficulty falling asleep, early morning awakening, and daytime fatigue are common. Alternatively, some patients during the depressive phase complain of excessive sleep, difficulty waking up, and excessive daytime somnolence. Disturbing dreams may also be a feature of sleep. Upon treatment, most sleep problems will end but insomnia can persist and continue to be troublesome.

What is sleep-related eating disorder?

This disorder is also called nocturnal binge-eating disorder. The person with the disorder experiences episodes of involuntary eating and drinking during the night, often (like sleepwalkers) with little recollection of their behavior. However, some sufferers appear to be very alert and can recollect what happened in the morning. Generally, high-calorie foods (carbohydrates and fats) are eaten. Often, food is consumed in odd combinations or is toxic or inedible. An example is a glass of soft drink mixed with dog biscuits. Usually sufferers don't have an appetite in the morning and can feel bloated. Weight gain is common.

Are there any sleep problems associated with anorexia nervosa or bulimia nervosa?

When weight is subnormal, the patient usually sleeps less. However, a complaint of insomnia is rare since the time is used by the patient for other activities, such as exercise. Binge eating can result in increased amounts of sleep and if it occurs at night, usually results in the person sleeping through the early part of the day. Sleep walking seems more common among people with eating disorders but this has not been systematically studied.

Sleep and seasonal affective disorder (SAD)

Q What is SAD?

SAD, or seasonal affective disorder, is a recurrent disturbance of mood occurring in winter or when light levels are naturally low. We all feel better when the sun is shining. On days that are gloomy, overcast, or rainy, we tend to feel less enthusiastic about life and tend to spend more time indoors. We even have a tendency to socialize less and to do less work. So when winter with its short days and long dark nights comes along, many of us feel a drop in enthusiasm for life and for getting out. If the condition is mild (subclinical SAD), it is referred to as the "winter blues" but when it is more severe and associated with major depression, then SAD is the appropriate term.

Q How common is SAD?

Approximately 2 in 100 people living in northern Canada, the northern US, and northern Europe get SAD and it is estimated that about 1 in 10 people suffer from subclinical SAD ("winter blues"). People who have grown up in tropical countries or have lived there for long periods of time may also be more susceptible to developing SAD once they move to a country that has a winter with low levels of light. SAD is very rare in people who live within 30 degrees north and south of the equator, because days and nights in winter and summer are almost always equivalent in length and the natural light levels are consistently strong and bright.

SYMPTOMS OF SEASONAL AFFECTIVE DISORDER

Symptoms of SAD are present during winter months when natural light levels are low and disappear in spring and/or summer. A diagnosis of SAD is made when symptoms are experienced over 2 or more winters and are not related to any other causes of depression, low mood, or other metabolic disturbances or illness.

Sleep problems: oversleeping; difficulty staying awake during the day; early morning waking; disturbed sleep

Mood: depression; anxiety; feelings of low self-esteem and self-worth; irritability: feeling inappropriately teary; suicidal; unable to cope with everyday stress; feeling tense

Eating: overeating; carbohydrate cravings; weight gain; bulimia (eating large amounts of food and then vomiting)

Energy levels: low energy levels; feelings of fatigue and lethargy

Social problems: avoiding social contact; irritability and anger

Thought processes: difficulty concentrating; memory difficulties

Libido: reduced interest in sexual contact or physical closeness

Hormonal problems: irregular menstrual periods

Substance abuse: increased risk of alcohol or recreational drug abuse

Immune system: increased susceptibility to viral infections

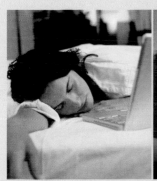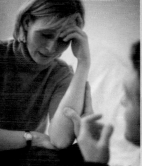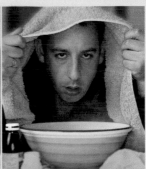

Q Who gets SAD?

SAD can begin at any age but generally develops between the ages of 18 and 30 years. It can sometimes be triggered by major life events, such as childbirth, a serious illness, or bereavement. SAD appears to be twice as common in women as in men, but this may be misleading since men are often less likely to want to admit to feelings of depression, anxiety, or an inability to cope with life.

Q What causes SAD?

Recognition of SAD as a distinct syndrome and scientific studies on its nature, consequences, and treatment have only been undertaken in the past 20 years. A number of factors lead to SAD but the exact cause is still unclear. However, it is known that the most important factor is the level of natural light required to trigger neurochemical and hormone production in the brain, via the hypothalamus. Brain serotonin levels are low in people depressed in winter and one factor for the symptoms of SAD could be inadequate production or effectiveness of serotonin.

Q Does melatonin play a role in SAD?

Melatonin levels (see p18) have been found to be high in people with SAD in winter with the levels normalizing in spring and summer. However, suppression of melatonin using bright light therapy doesn't cure all symptoms of SAD because it is only one potential mechanism leading to this disorder. Another theory used to explain some of the symptoms of SAD and its seasonality includes subtle changes or disruptions in the way the body clock works. A slowing down of the circadian rhythms may result from changes along any of the neural pathways from the suprachiasmatic nucleus to the hypothalamus.

LIGHT THERAPY

Light therapy (phototherapy) is one of the most effective treatments of SAD. It is effective in 4 out of 5 people within 3–5 days after treatment has commenced. Lightboxes can sometimes be obtained through a specialized sleep center and there are many companies that market lightboxes that can be used for SAD. Ask your sleep specialist or doctor for advice.

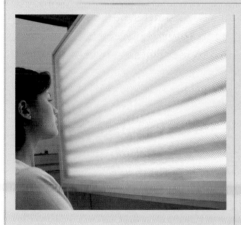

TREATMENT

Light treatment should start in the fall or when symptoms usually appear and continue on a daily basis until spring. The therapy comprises sitting near to or in front of a lightbox (about 2–3ft away) and allowing the light to shine on the eyes. Any device that blocks the passage of light to the retina, such as tinted lenses, should not be worn. Light therapy should be used from the early morning and through the day. However, it is best not to use it at night so that you still retain your natural melatonin secretion and can fall asleep.

EXPOSURE

Exposure to light should be undertaken from 30 minutes to several hours a day. Two hours a day is generally sufficient and the maximum recommended is 4. The light is not ordinary, but extremely bright light that is at least 20 times the intensity of ordinary domestic lighting. Occasionally, lightbox use can lead to headaches, irritability, or nausea. If this occurs, try to lessen exposure time. If problems persist, seek medical advice.

DOSAGE

The minimum dose of light intensity to treat SAD is 10,000 lux, whereas most domestic and office lighting (especially fluorescent lighting) delivers only 200–500 lux. A special lightbox must be used because some solar/suntan lamps and lightboxes emit too much UV light, which can be harmful to the eyes.

Q When does SAD occur?

In the Northern Hemisphere, SAD occurs between September and April and is generally most severe in the darkest months from December to February. A diagnosis of SAD can be made with confidence if symptoms occur over consecutive winters.

Q What happens in SAD?

Symptoms of SAD (see box, p105) are seasonal, so unlike a depressive illness it occurs only in winter. Most people with SAD have a gradual resolution of their symptoms as the days get longer in spring; some even have a short burst of mania and hyperactivity once spring arrives. But all the symptoms should disappear. In subclinical SAD, depression or anxiety are absent or mild. In the Northern Hemisphere, most people with subclinical SAD have their worst phases in the darkest months from December to February. Fatigue and eating or sleeping problems are typical of "winter blues" and symptoms last a shorter time.

Q How is SAD treated?

The most common and effective treatment for SAD is light therapy (see p107). Psychotherapy, counseling, and cognitive-behavioral therapy (see pp182–183 for all of these) can all be useful adjuncts to the treatment of SAD.

Q Can antidepressant medication help in the treatment of SAD?

If SAD is severe, medications to increase brain serotonin levels can help, and can be combined with light treatment (see p107) if necessary. Paroxetine, fluoxetine, and sertraline are examples of medications that improve serotonin balance and can be prescribed by your doctor. These medications usually take a few weeks to be effective.

Are there any permanent cures for SAD?

Relocating to a country close to the equator is the only known "cure." A winter break to a sunnier region or even skiing (bright light reflected off the snow) can be therapeutic. However, if you then return to darkness, your symptoms of SAD will recur.

What can my family and friends do to help me cope with SAD?

Information and understanding are important to make living together easier. A supportive family member, friend, or partner can encourage you to stick to therapy and make helpful lifestyle changes (see box below). Self-help groups and websites provide support and information, too (see p184).

WHAT ELSE CAN I DO TO HELP PREVENT SAD?

- Try to get outdoors during the darker winter months, especially in the middle of the day, although this does not necessarily cure SAD.

- Try to work next to a window with natural light.

- Paint your walls white or in pale colors to enhance brightness inside your home.

- Keep winter time as stress-free as possible. This can be difficult at certain times (such as when there are family get-togethers at Thanksgiving and Christmas); avoid over-commitments.

- Plan life-changing events, such as a big move or changing jobs, for the summer months if possible.

- Get active—exercise is known to improve mood. Activities that get you out in natural light, such as a lunchtime walk, may be particularly helpful, but any type of exercise brings benefits.

- Pamper yourself. Relaxation techniques and pampering therapies (massage, aromatherapy, etc.) can be of help.

- Keep your diet healthy—try to balance your cravings for carbohydrates with plenty of vegetables and proteins.

Myth "Sleep needs decline with age"

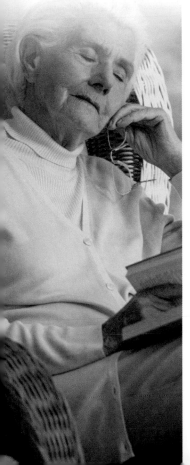

Truth This is a common misconception. The actual amount of sleep we need changes very little with aging. What does change is the pattern of our sleep, in that as we grow old we experience less slow wave sleep (especially men) and slightly less REM sleep. Healthy older adults tend to sleep well. Trouble falling asleep at night or excessive drowsiness during the day is neither normal nor inevitable in old age.

How aging affects sleep

What causes sleep disturbances in older age?

A number of factors can result in poor sleep in older age. First, poor sleep hygiene habits are difficult to change. Second, a medical or mood disorder that adversely affects sleep becomes more likely and the medications to treat it may also lead to sleep disturbances. Thirdly, the incidence of primary sleep disorders like sleep apnea increase and can contribute to sleep disturbance (this includes a bed partner who can affect your quality of sleep). And lastly, aging affects our bladders, circadian rhythms, hormone secretion, and body temperature so it can lead to less refreshing and more disrupted sleep.

Can lifestyle factors influence sleep in aging?

Yes. Evidence from a number of studies suggests that sleep difficulties are greater in the older person who has little or no exposure to natural light, has a poor diet, does not exercise, and is not mentally stimulated. This means that as far as you are able, you should keep yourself active, involved in life and with others (family, friends, volunteer activities, or work), keep up an exercise routine suited to your physical needs, and eat a healthy and balanced diet.

The older I get, the earlier I tend to wake up in the morning – is this normal?

As your circadian rhythm changes with age, you tend to feel more tired toward the early evening, thus bringing your bedtime forward. When this occurs, you tend to wake up earlier, so the cycle continues. There is nothing wrong with this, unless your bedtime has advanced to the degree that you are suffering from advanced sleep phase syndrome (see p77) and it is impairing your day-to-day functioning.

HOW DOES SLEEP CHANGE AS WE AGE?

The observations that have been made about sleep at various stages of our lives are summarized below. As we get older, we have less slow wave sleep (stages 3 and 4) and a reduction in the amount of REM sleep during the night. The amount of time spent awake after going to bed also increases—it may take longer to fall asleep, and wake up more often during the night and earlier in the morning. The amount of time we spend asleep decreases only slightly.

	Infants	Young adults	Elderly
Time spent awake after sleep onset	> 5%	> 5%	10–20%
Sleep efficiency	< 90%	< 90%	80–85%
Stage 1 amount	Inactive sleep	2–8%	4–10%
Stage 2 amount	Inactive sleep	45–55%	35–45%
Stages 3 & 4 amount	Inactive sleep	13–23%	5–18%
REM sleep amount	50%	20–25%	15–20%
Time of REM/NREM cycle	45–60 mins	90–110 mins	90–110 mins
Total sleep time	45–60 mins	7–8 hours	7 hours

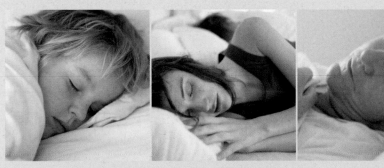

What are the changes that lead to sleep disruption in older age?

As we age, the body's production of growth hormone (produced during slow wave sleep), sex hormones, and melatonin begins to decline. The changes, especially in growth hormone levels, coincide with the reduction in slow wave sleep. Changes in temperature regulation also occur. Serum cortisol levels rise with age and the evening dip is not as pronounced as in younger people. This change in cortisol levels is associated with the observed reduction in REM sleep with age. Levels of inflammatory neurochemicals (cytokines) in the bloodstream also tend to be more elevated in elderly as compared to younger people who sleep poorly. Some of these cytokines can cause symptoms of daytime sleepiness and fatigue.

What are the most common primary sleep disorders?

The most common sleep disorders in the elderly are insomnia, sleep apnea, restless legs syndrome, and advanced sleep phase syndrome.

Is it normal to be tired during the day in old age?

No. Although stamina, endurance levels, and organ function start to decline from about 30 years of age, if you are otherwise healthy, sleep well, take no medication, and have a balanced lifestyle, there is no reason to be tired.

What about all the pills I'm on—could they be affecting my sleep?

Many medications can disrupt sleep. A list of commonly prescribed drugs is provided on p44. The time at which you take medication can also affect sleep, so talk to your doctor if you think that a drug is causing sleep disturbances. Many elderly people take a wide variety of prescribed drugs for various ailments—if you are unsure why you are on certain medications and what they should be doing, discuss this with your doctor. Don't be shy about discussing your health with the appropriate professional.

Q Is it normal to nap in old age?

This is a difficult question with no precise answer yet. At present it is thought that the lightening of sleep at night results from a reduced drive to sleep and the corollary of this is an increased urge to nap during the day. However, studies in people who age successfully (without medical disease, psychiatric disorders, or sleep disorders) show that even well into their 80s they have no increase in daytime sleepiness requiring naps. So, if you feel excessively sleepy or tired during the day, don't let anyone tell you that it is just due to old age. Daytime sleepiness in old age is usually the result of many different factors working together to cause sleep difficulties and disruption.

Q My bladder keeps me up all night —what can I do about it?

As your bladder ages, it is less likely to retain as much urine over longer periods of time. It is important to discuss your symptoms with a medical professional and sometimes a specialist (urologist) who can help diagnose and manage your problem. Men who get up to urinate during the night and have problems with stream or with dribbling should have their prostate checked; most men experience these symptoms due to enlargement of the prostate gland. Tell your doctor if you have a burning or stinging sensation when urinating and ask about Kegel exercises and medications for erectile dysfunction.

Q What can I do to minimize sleep disruption?

Reduce the amount of fluid you drink in the evening and just before going to bed. If you are on a diuretic medication, take it in the morning and the last dose at lunchtime. If you have a primary bladder problem, make sure you have comfortable incontinence pads. Sometimes the need to urinate during the night is associated with a sleep disorder such as sleep apnea.

Sleep and drugs

Which drugs affect sleep?

A large number of medications can affect both quality and quantity of sleep. Medications can also alter the proportions of REM and NREM sleep that we experience. Some commonly prescribed drugs have been discussed in previous chapters. If you think that a medication that you have been prescribed might be affecting your sleep patterns, sleep quality, or sleep content, seek medical advice from a doctor.

How does marijuana use affect sleep?

The short-term use of marijuana causes minimal sleep disruption, with a slight reduction in REM sleep. However, long-term use of marijuana leads to long-term suppression of slow wave sleep.

What about the effects of other illegal drugs?

Cocaine acts as a stimulant so it reduces your perceived need for sleep, as do amphetamines. MDMA (ecstasy) has very similar effects and therein lies its danger—because people often don't realize how tired or dehydrated they are, they keep going past the limit of their endurance. Long-term use of stimulant medication can result in changes in sleep patterns that may be very difficult to treat. GHB (gamma hydroxybutyrate), a "date rape drug," can cause sleepiness and, in high doses, can reduce the drive to breathe, potentially leading to respiratory arrest and death if untreated. Other date rape drugs are very strong sedatives from the benzodiazepine class that can induce sleepiness and also reduce the drive to breathe. Morphine and heroin have the same effect.

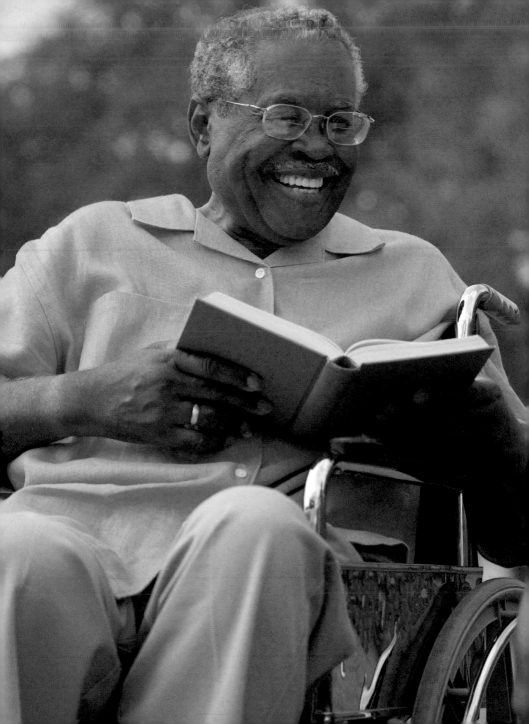

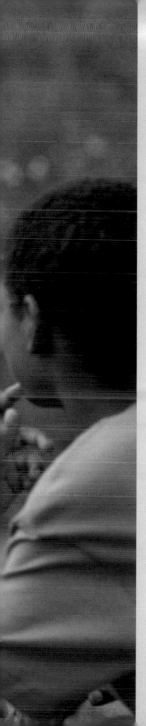

Sleep and neurological problems

Sleep can be affected by diseases of the nervous system and muscles. Muscle problems (such as myotonic dystrophy or myasthenia gravis) can cause breathing problems that disrupt sleep if they are severe enough. Diseases affecting the brain and its development play havoc with sleep needs, sleep itself, and may also be associated with sleep disorders such as narcolepsy and REM-behavior disorder.

Common neurological diseases

Q **I have Parkinson's disease. How does this affect my sleep?**

It is common to have sleep problems in all forms of parkinsonism but you should discuss them with your doctor. The problems experienced include insomnia, decreased ability to move at night, and REM-behavior disorder with sudden, sometimes violent movement and talking or shouting. Sleep problems increase as Parkinson's disease worsens. Daytime drowsiness becomes more common; some people have sleep attacks during the day. Breathing can also be disturbed in Parkinson's disease.

Q **Why can sleep be disrupted in Parkinson's disease?**

There are many different causes of poor sleep in Parkinson's disease. Problems with sleep-wake control mechanisms due to neurochemical imbalances can result in fragmented sleep and a reduction in REM sleep. Slowed movement and rigidity can lead to a reduction in the number of normal body shifts during sleep. This in turn may lead to discomfort and awakenings, as well as problems with getting up to use the bathroom at night. There is an increased association in Parkinson's disease with periodic leg movements, tremors, and jerking movements due to medication, all of which can lead to increased awakenings. Depression and anxiety can result in problems falling asleep and staying asleep, as well as early morning awakenings. Dementia occurring in Parkinson's disease can result in episodes of confusion at night. Sleep-disordered breathing may also occur.

How can sleep disturbances in Parkinson's disease be managed?

Sleep disturbances in Parkinson's disease need to be managed in conjunction with your doctor. Management involves good control of symptoms and careful use of your medications. Many of the medications used to treat Parkinson's disease can also have adverse effects on sleep and can worsen some sleep disturbances. Causes of insomnia need to be investigated and managed as described in pp53–54. Symptoms of sleep apnea or significant snoring need to be taken seriously, investigated by a sleep specialist, and treated. Stimulant medications may be useful in people who experience sleep attacks. However, any medication changes or adjustments should only be made after you are thoroughly assessed by your treating doctor or neurologist.

What sort of sleep disturbances occur in stroke?

Strokes can affect any part of the brain and lead to problems with sleep and daytime symptoms such as fatigue. Depending on which part of the brain is affected various breathing abnormalities can emerge which may require treatment. About 2 to 4 in 10 patients have increased sleep needs, excessive daytime sleepiness, and insomnia. Fatigue is found in up to 3 of 4 patients. Sometimes people with stroke develop parasomnias and may lose their perception of time. Disruptions in the circadian rhythm can also occur.

Does stroke result in sleep-disordered breathing?

About 6 to 7 in 10 people who have a stroke develop sleep-disordered breathing after the stroke. In many cases, this will settle with time. It has also been found that many people who have a stroke have had symptoms of sleep apnea prior to the stroke, but whether this caused their problems is not yet known with certainty.

Q Why can sleep be disrupted in stroke?

Stroke may cause sleep-wake disturbances for many reasons. The most important is the damage to the brain tissue and the neurochemical pathways that occurs directly as a result of the stroke. Other factors can be caused by the hospital environment. These may include noise, too much light, and intensive medical monitoring. Sleep fragmentation can result from sleep-disordered breathing, infections, heart problems, lung disease, seizures, fever, and medications. Mood change in the form of depression and anxiety can affect the sleep-wake cycle, as does the psychological stress of coping with the stroke.

Q I've had brain surgery—why am I so sleepy?

There can be many factors contributing to fatigue after such major surgery, including damage to the brain tissue and disruption of neuronal pathways, however subtle, that regulate the sleep-wake cycle. Fatigue is normal after any major surgery. It may take many months to overcome this. Of course, sleep-disordered breathing or another primary sleep disorder should be treated. Some of the anticonvulsant medications which are used after surgery can also contribute to sleepiness and increased fatigue.

Q My partner has dementia—how does this affect sleep?

There are many different causes of dementia, not just Alzheimer's disease, although this is the most common. The types of sleep problems that people with dementia have tend to fall into a number of categories. These include: insomnia, excessive daytime sleepiness, changes to the circadian rhythm, and excessive movement during the night, including REM-behavior disorder and restless legs syndrome.

What other sleep problems do people with dementia have?

One of the most noticeable and distressing sleep problems in people with dementia (most commonly Alzheimer's disease) is nocturnal wandering, agitation, and delirium. This is called sun-downing. People with dementia may also have problems with sleep-disordered breathing, and other illnesses can contribute to problems with sleep.

What can be done about sleep problems in dementia?

As with all sleep disturbances, the appropriate treatments outlined on pp35–42 should be tried first before resorting to medication. Eliminate caffeine, alcohol, and disruptive influences on the sleeping environment. We often ignore very basic factors that can be distressing to someone who can no longer communicate well. These include a full bladder, constipation, heat or cold due to an inappropriate environment or clothing, pain from infections or pressure sores, inadequate exercise during the day, or a disruptive bedroom environment. Sometimes a night light next to the bed can be useful for orientation and may reduce anxiety. There are many effective medications for treating sleep disorders associated with dementia and your doctor can advise you about which ones you can try.

I have post-polio syndrome—how can this affect my sleep?

Many people with post-polio syndrome experience an increasing weakness of the muscles that control breathing, especially the rib cage muscles and sometimes even the diaphragm, as they age. This can lead to breathing problems at night with a drop in blood oxygen levels and a rise in carbon dioxide levels. This in turn can lead to symptoms of increased daytime fatigue, morning headaches, and reduced appetite. Poor sleep and fatigue can make muscular problems worse. Treatment of nocturnal breathing problems was discussed on pp84–89.

Myth "People with intellectual disability can't be treated for sleep problems"

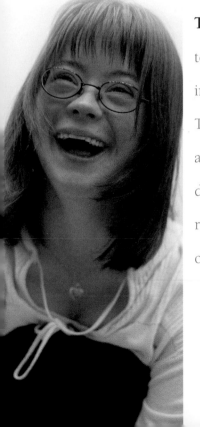

Truth This is untrue. Behavioral measures to deal with sleep problems in people with intellectual disability can be very effective. The treatment for primary sleep disorders such as sleep apnea, narcolepsy, or circadian rhythm disorders may be slightly more complex, but can result in enormous improvements in the quality of life and health.

Adults with intellectual disability

What is intellectual disability?

"Intellectual disability" (ID) is used to describe a person over the age of 5 who has significantly below-average general intellectual functioning. The person must also show deficits in day-to-day behavior that have become obvious between the ages of 1 and 18 years. Intellectual function is assessed by intelligence tests to give an intelligence quotient (IQ). An average IQ is considered to be 100, while a below-average IQ is one below 70. However, this assessment alone is not sufficient. Tests of day-to-day functioning may reveal more closely how independent someone is and whether simple tasks need to be done in the context of education, support, and training. About 3 in 100 people have mild or greater (moderate, severe, profound) intellectual disability.

What are the causes of intellectual disability?

There are various causes of intellectual disability. About 60 percent of causes of ID are prenatal. These include chromosome errors (such as Down syndrome) and single gene errors, developmental disorders, and intrauterine problems (toxins, infections). Factors that can occur around birth include cerebral damage and hemorrhage. Infections, accidents, and abuse can also contribute to the development of ID. The most common types of ID include autistic disorders, Down syndrome, Prader–Willi syndrome, fragile X syndrome, and familial intellectual disability.

Q What sleep disorders do people with ID have?

Intellectual disability (ID) is common within our society but the needs of people with disability are often overlooked. Caregivers and parents often do not receive the support necessary to look after children, let alone adults, with intellectual disability. The health needs of people with ID are specialized. One aspect of ID that is often overlooked is sleep. People with ID can have primary sleep disorders that can lead to behavioral disturbances and sleepiness just as in those without ID. Sleep hygiene and behavioral changes with regard to sleep can be more challenging to treat in this group of patients, but if successful, can be extremely rewarding as everybody's quality of life is improved.

Q Why is sleep important for people with ID?

People with ID generally have a large number of other disabilities and conditions to deal with, so a good night's sleep is essential to their well-being just like anybody else's. The literature on sleep disturbance in adults with ID is sparse, but the prevalence of sleep disorders in children with ID is up to 4 times higher than in children who are developing normally, which can exacerbate other problems.

Q How can sleep be impaired in people with ID?

Physical problems or disabilities that can cause pain, discomfort, or frustration can lead to impairment of sleep in people with ID. Other factors such as problems with eyesight or hearing, medication effects, epilepsy, and mood disorders can affect sleep in people with ID just like in other people. People with ID can also suffer from all the primary sleep disorders mentioned on pp50–81, such as sleep apnea, narcolepsy, and restless legs syndrome, as well as developing insomnia.

What are the most common sleep disorders in people with ID?

The most common sleep disorders in people with ID are insomnia, excessive daytime sleepiness, and daytime napping. Night waking is also very common. In Down syndrome, sleep apnea is very common and often goes unrecognized and untreated. Children with ID, especially with autism, often have problems with settling at night.

How do people with ID report sleep problems?

Often people with ID will not directly report a sleep problem and rely on the observations of an astute parent or caregiver to pick up on excessive daytime sleepiness, night time discomfort, or abnormal sleep behaviors. Fatigue can manifest itself in a variety of ways including mood disturbances (depression), aggression, noncompliance with instructions, hyperactivity, self-injury, screaming, and socially inappropriate behavior.

How will a caregiver/parent know that a person with ID has a sleep disturbance?

Parents and caregivers often accept sleep disturbances and abnormal sleep patterns in people with ID as part of the person's condition and do little about it. However, this can result in long-term harm to the person's health and impair quality of life. If you witness abnormal behavior during sleep such as snoring, breathing pauses, and restlessness, it is important to bring it to the attention of the doctor or health professional involved in the care of the person with ID.

Can mood disorders disrupt sleep in people with ID?

Depression and anxiety can lead to sleep disturbances and cause a vicious cycle of problems, so it is important these are recognized and reported. People with ID often show behavior problems when in reality they may have an underlying medical problem causing their distress.

Q Can blindness make sleep patterns worse in someone with ID?

Yes, depending on how severe the blindness is. In people who do not have any light transmission to their suprachiasmatic nucleus (a small cluster of light-responsive cells), there can be significant problems with circadian rhythms and sleep. Treatment includes behavioral measures as outlined on pp35–42, especially keeping a regular bedtime and waking time. Melatonin has proven to be a very effective treatment in these disorders. If you think someone has sleep disturbances due to blindness, discuss this with his or her doctor.

Q Do people with Down syndrome have sleep apnea?

Sleep apnea is a common problem in people with Down syndrome. The reported prevalence ranges from 31–63 percent in children with Down syndrome. The prevalence in the adult population with Down syndrome is currently unknown but is also presumed to be high.

Q Why do people with Down syndrome get sleep apnea?

There are a number of physical attributes in people with Down syndrome that predispose them to developing sleep apnea. These include a small midface (low-set cheekbones), the tendency to have a small jaw which is also backset, a narrow palate, narrow nasal passages, and a narrow throat. They are more prone to blockage of the nasal passages at birth (this can be fixed at birth and even later in life), a broad skull, small larynx, a relatively large tongue compared to the size of their mouth, enlarged tonsils and adenoids, increased secretions, low thyroid levels, and general floppiness of the muscles. People with Down syndrome also tend to be less active and put on weight very easily, which can predispose them to obesity and result in problems with sleep-disordered breathing at night.

What are the consequences of untreated sleep apnoea in Down syndrome?

As in everybody with sleep apnea, narrowing of the upper airway during the night can result in prolonged breathing pauses, which can cause blood oxygen levels to drop with concurrent rise of carbon dioxide. This can worsen problems such as pulmonary hypertension and may even lead to heart failure. People with Down syndrome have a greater risk of developing heart problems and elevated right heart pressures. The daytime effects of disrupted sleep can also manifest as abnormal levels of sleepiness, learning difficulties, behavioral disturbances, depression, irritability, paranoia, and personality changes. Sleep problems can also worsen cognitive function in these people.

How are sleep disturbances managed in an adult with ID?

If you think that someone with ID may have a sleep problem resulting in a disturbed sleep-wake cycle, excessive daytime sleepiness, or changes in behavior patterns or mood, then you and the person with ID must make the doctor aware of this. Primary sleep disorders can be assessed in a sleep laboratory or equipment may be available to take home if the person with ID is more comfortable with this—something you need to discuss with your sleep specialist.

Can behavioral treatments help?

Behavioral treatments are available and are highly effective (examples include reward systems and desensitization). They may require a bit of concentration and persistence on behalf of the caregiver to implement at times, but, when successful, can be extremely rewarding for all concerned. However, the most important aspect of treating a sleep disorder or behavioral disorder due to poor sleep lies in recognizing it.

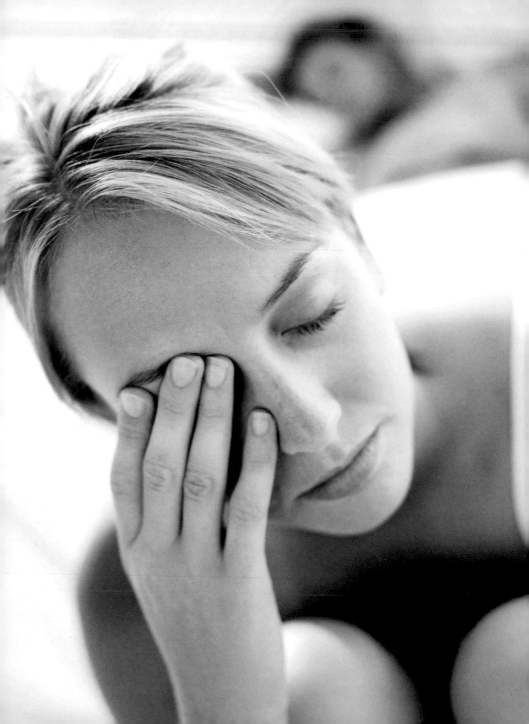

Women
and sleep

Sleep patterns in women change throughout their lives and are influenced strongly by the female hormones, namely estrogen and progesterone. Menstruation, pregnancy, and menopause all have a unique impact on the quantity and quality of sleep experienced by women. They also affect the incidence and prevalence of primary sleep disorders in women.

Sleep differences between the sexes

Q Are there any differences in sleep quality and/or quantity between men and women?

Throughout life, there are small differences in sleep patterns between men and women, which may not be very significant but become more evident with age. The hypothalamus responds to estrogen and progesterone (the female sex hormones), which may influence sleep and circadian rhythms. Women are more likely to suffer from and report insomnia. Prior to menopause, women are less likely to suffer from sleep apnea than after menopause, when the incidence of sleep apnea among women increases, probably due to increased weight.

Q Are there differences in sleep regulation between men and women?

It is well known that there are gender differences in brain structure, regulation, and function between men and women. For instance, parts of the hypothalamus are larger in men than women; growth hormone production is higher in women than in men. Although research on sleep and circadian rhythms has been limited, there is some evidence of differences in sleep regulation throughout life between men and women (see box, p131).

Q Are the differences in sleep patterns between men and women very significant?

In healthy young adults, differences in sleep quality and quantity are very subtle. These can become more obvious if there is a challenge to the body, such as sleep deprivation, disease, stress, drugs, or major depression. Variation in hormone levels vary during the menstrual cycle and, in menopause, can also affect responses to stress and lead to changes in sleep. Research is still continuing in this area.

SLEEP DIFFERENCES BETWEEN MEN AND WOMEN

The table below summarizes the differences in sleep between men and women throughout life. Since these findings are based on only a few studies, they may not prove to be entirely correct in the long term. Probably, the most consistent difference overall is that men have greater age-related changes in sleep than women; the quantity and quality of sleep in women stay slightly more constant throughout life.

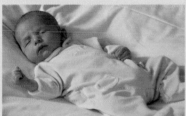

INFANCY

Boys sleep less and wake more often

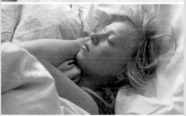

CHILDHOOD

Girls sleep for a longer time

Earlier bedtime in girls

Boys have more severe sleep problems

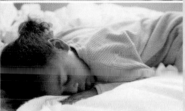

ADOLESCENCE

Girls sleep for a longer time

Girls wake up earlier

Girls are sleepier

Boys wake more often

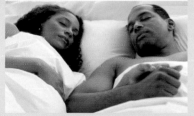

ADULTHOOD

Men have more Stage 1 sleep

Women have more slow wave sleep

Men wake up more often

Women tend to report worse sleep

Sleep and menstruation

Q How does the menstrual cycle affect sleep?

The hormones estrogen and progesterone play a role in regulating the menstrual cycle and also, through their additional functions relating to the brain, influence other processes like sleep and circadian rhythms. Changes that occur in women's bodies during the menstrual cycle can affect sleep. Many women report 2–3 days of disrupted sleep during each cycle. Some report more sleep in the premenstrual period, while others report insomnia. Factors like stress, mood, illness, medication, diet, and sleep environment can also affect sleep at this time. Menstrual cycles are usually 25–35 days long.

Q What is sleep like before ovulation?

Day 1 of the menstrual cycle is identified as the first day of bleeding (menses). Bleeding usually continues for about 5 days. During this time, many women sleep less and feel less comfortable during their sleep time. Those who suffer from menstrual cramping and pain obviously spend more time awake due to pain than those who don't, have greater movement activity during sleep, and experience more stage 1 (lighter) sleep and less REM sleep. When bleeding stops and estrogen levels start to rise, women may experience more REM sleep.

Q Does sleep change at the time of ovulation?

Around day 14, ovulation (release of an egg from the ovary) occurs. Estrogen levels in the blood peak just before ovulation. During this time, there are no real changes in sleep quality or quantity, but there may be subtle differences in the amount of REM and slow wave sleep in women who have ovulated successfully.

THE MENSTRUAL CYCLE

By convention, the menstrual cycle is represented as lasting 28 days to show the changes that occur throughout the cycle. The first day of bleeding (menses) is day 1. Ovulation (release of the egg from the ovary) is day 14.

The cycle is thus divided into 2 phases. The first phase of the cycle (prior to ovulation) is the follicular phase. During this stage, as the egg starts to grow in the follicle, the levels of estrogen are high. The high estrogen levels cause a surge in luteinizing hormone (LH), which controls fertility and is the trigger for ovulation.

During the second half of the cycle (the luteal phase), the levels of progesterone are much higher than oestrogen levels and resting body temperature may rise by as much as 1°F (½°C). If there is no fertilization and implantation of the egg during the luteal phase, the hormonal levels eventually drop drastically and bleeding commences.

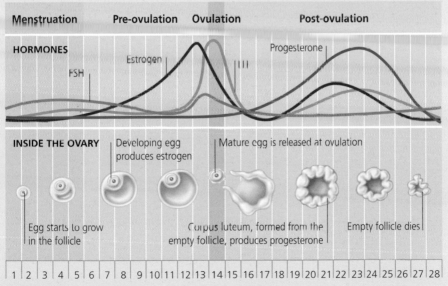

Menstruation   **Pre-ovulation**   **Ovulation**   **Post-ovulation**

HORMONES

Estrogen

FSH

Progesterone

INSIDE THE OVARY   Developing egg produces estrogen   Mature egg is released at ovulation

Egg starts to grow in the follicle   Corpus luteum, formed from the empty follicle, produces progesterone   Empty follicle dies

| 1 | 2 | 3 | 4 | 5 | 6 | 7 | 8 | 9 | 10 | 11 | 12 | 13 | 14 | 15 | 16 | 17 | 18 | 19 | 20 | 21 | 22 | 23 | 24 | 25 | 26 | 27 | 28 |

Days of cycle

Q What happens to sleep after ovulation?

If the egg is fertilized after its release, pregnancy will ensue. Otherwise, this stage of the cycle is dominated by the hormone progesterone. If fertilization does not occur, hormone levels drop dramatically and menstruation occurs. Some women may find it difficult to sleep during this time. Others suffer from premenstrual syndrome (PMS), with bloating, irritability, headaches, moodiness, and abdominal cramps. All of these may affect the quality of sleep. Some women may experience drastic changes to their sleep including excessive sleep, insomnia for a couple of nights prior to their period, or significant daytime sleepiness. Depending on the severity and whether the problem is long- or short-term, this can be classified as a sleep disorder.

Q What can I do to improve my sleep, especially premenstrually?

The general lifestyle tips discussed on p29 will be useful to you. If you suffer from premenstrual syndrome or have severe mood changes (depression, anger, and irritability that affect normal functioning), you should seek medical advice. Apart from modifying lifestyle factors, there are some effective medications that can be very useful in controlling symptoms. Sometimes going on an oral contraceptive may help considerably.

Q How do oral contraceptives affect ovulation?

Many women take oral contraceptives for long periods of time to regulate their menstrual cycles and to control fertility. Oral contraceptives are combined formulations of low-dose progestin and synthetic estrogen and suppress the body's own production of these hormones. They, thus, prevent ovulation (production of an egg from the ovaries), interrupting the normal course of the cycle.

Can oral contraceptives have an impact on sleep?

Oral contraceptives affect body temperature regulation and can affect sleep. Body temperatures are consistently raised throughout the cycle, unlike in women who are not on the pill. Secretion of melatonin may also be affected although the research evidence is currently still under review. Women on oral contraceptives have more stage 2 sleep and less slow wave sleep, the deep sleep that is thought to be restful and restorative. They are likely to have more REM sleep than women not on oral contraceptives.

What is polycystic ovarian syndrome and how does it affect sleep?

Polycystic ovarian syndrome (PCOS) is a disorder in hormone production in which some of the ovarian cells produce too much androgen (male hormones). PCOS affects up to 4 in 100 women of child-bearing age and results in disrupted and irregular periods, weight gain, a tendency to develop diabetes, and excessive body hair. The risks for developing high blood pressure and heart problems are also increased. With regard to sleep, women with PCOS have a higher risk of developing sleep-disordered breathing and sleep apnea (probably due to weight gain) and are more likely to report symptoms of excessive daytime sleepiness. PCOS is usually treated by a specialist in hormones (endocrinologist).

Does shift-work affect the menstrual cycle?

Shift-work can disrupt circadian rhythms in hormone production. The reproductive/sex hormones are also affected. Studies show that women shift-workers have more irregular menstrual cycles, painful menstruation, and longer menstrual cycles than women who are non-shift workers. Stress probably plays a large part in affecting the secretion of hormones from the pituitary gland that then regulate the production of sex hormones.

Sleep and pregnancy

Q How does pregnancy affect sleep?

Pregnancy is very demanding for any woman and is a time of great sleep disruption. Many factors contribute to this: hormonal changes, the growing fetus, discomfort (vomiting, heartburn, cramps, pressure on the bladder), mood changes, and anxiety related to delivery. Some women develop sleep disorders, such as restless legs syndrome and sleep apnea, for the first time. After the birth, the new baby's demands take precedence over the mother's need for sleep.

IMPROVING SLEEP DURING PREGNANCY

- Ensure that you have a high intake of folate, iron, and vitamin B_{12} before and during pregnancy.
- Exercise regularly and control weight.
- Keep fluid intake high, but try to cut down before bedtime to ease the stress on your bladder.
- If heartburn is a problem, sleep with the head of your bed elevated, or use a few pillows.
- Eating small meals during the day and avoiding spicy, fatty, or fried food may reduce acid reflux and help with nausea, especially in the first trimester.
- Schedule naps during the day, to help with daytime fatigue.

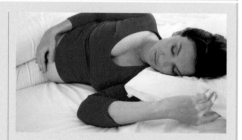

- As your pregnancy progresses, adjust your bedding accordingly. Special pregnancy pillows and support pillows may make sleeping more comfortable.
- In the third trimester, try to sleep on your left side (rather than your back) to allow for improved blood flow to the fetus, uterus, and kidneys.

Do women snore more during pregnancy?

About 1 in 3 women will snore during pregnancy, 15–20 percent of them for the first time. If this is severe enough, it may be associated with higher blood pressure during pregnancy, and 1 in 10 pregnant snorers develop preeclampsia (high blood pressure, fluid retention, and protein in urine during pregnancy). Significant snoring during pregnancy should be assessed by a doctor.

Can women develop sleep apnea during pregnancy?

Obese women who are pregnant and women who gain excessive weight while pregnant are at a higher risk of developing sleep apnea. A drop in blood oxygen levels at night is associated with potential complications for the baby. It is important that overweight women and women who gain a lot of weight during pregnancy should be assessed by a doctor for evidence of sleep apnea.

Do women experience restless leg syndrome (RLS) during pregnancy?

The other major sleep disorder that can occur during pregnancy is restless legs syndrome (RLS) and leg cramp. About 15–25 percent of women develop RLS during pregnancy in association with iron deficiency and women with low folate levels are also at risk. Although RLS will end after delivery, it is an additional stressor during pregnancy and can disrupt sleep, so make sure that you have adequate iron, folate, and vitamin B_{12} levels in your blood before and during pregnancy.

How does sleep change after delivery?

Up to 4 in 5 women experience "baby blues" 3 to 5 days after delivery. The blues generally don't last longer that about 2 weeks, but 1 in 5 women develop postpartum depression. Postpartum depression can occur any time within 6 months of delivery and, like any mood disorder, it can result in severe sleep disruption.

Sleep patterns during pregnancy

Sleep patterns change throughout pregnancy, largely as a result of the enormous physical changes that take place as the fetus grows, but also partly due to hormonal changes that occur.

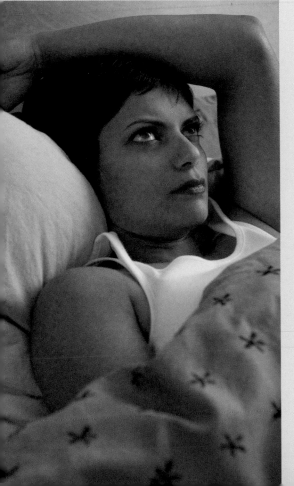

SLEEP DURING THE FIRST TRIMESTER

The first trimester is the period from conception to 3 months. During this time, the high levels of progesterone in the body have a sleep-inducing and sedating effect on the brain. Progesterone also increases the need to urinate due to the effect it has on the smooth muscle in the bladder. Women often experience more sleep difficulty during the night due to an increased need to go to the bathroom. Many women experience daytime sleepiness and fatigue during this time. Nausea and vomiting is not just limited to "morning sickness" but can also occur in the evening. There is a greater tendency to sleep longer than prior to pregnancy, but there is less slow wave sleep during this time.

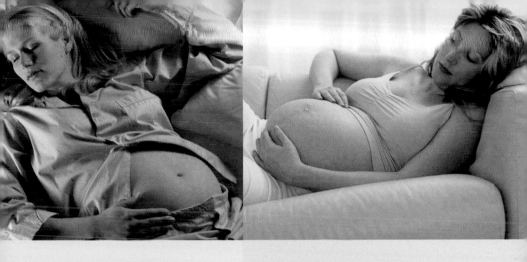

SLEEP DURING THE SECOND TRIMESTER

The second trimester of pregnancy is the period from the fourth to the sixth month. Progesterone levels continue to rise during this period but more slowly. Many women experience a great improvement in their sleep quality and quantity during this period and report more daytime energy. The growing fetus moves above the bladder and the need to urinate decreases. However, many women start to snore at this stage, probably because of the effects of estrogen on blood vessels, resulting in nasal congestion. During this time, there is an increased risk of developing sleep apnea and also high blood pressure, so you must be carefully monitored by your doctor. There is less slow wave sleep than prior to pregnancy and more time is spent awake during the night.

SLEEP DURING THE THIRD TRIMESTER

The third trimester is the period from the seventh to the ninth month. Progesterone levels are at their peak during this time. Women report the most sleep difficulties during this stage of pregnancy. Sleep disturbances are very common and are caused by a wide variety of factors, including leg cramps, heartburn, nasal congestion, and an increased need to urinate. The baby's movements can also disturb sleep. In the last few weeks of pregnancy, many women find achieving a comfortable sleeping position difficult. This can lead to increased daytime fatigue and sleepiness. Breast tenderness, shortness of breath, and irregular uterine contractions can also affect sleep adversely. Overall, more time is spent awake and there is less slow wave sleep.

Early stages of motherhood

Q What sort of sleep disruptions occur after pregnancy?

Unsurprisingly, women experience more awakenings at night after delivery (for feeding of the baby), although this tends to settle after the first month. Many mothers find daytime naps are a good way to compensate for this disruption in sleep during the night. For first-time mothers, the first 3–6 weeks after delivery are very tiring and fatigue levels remain high for 3 months (higher than prior to pregnancy). There is a high proportion of slow wave sleep after pregnancy related largely to the production of the hormone prolactin responsible for "letting down milk."

Q How can I ensure that I get enough sleep in the early stages of looking after my baby?

Initially it will be difficult for you to have uninterrupted sleep during the night. But the good news is that once your baby has a regular sleep-wake pattern (by about 6 months), things will start to return to normal. To combat fatigue, make sure that you eat well—iron levels are low after pregnancy and this can make you feel more tired. Scheduling a nap when the baby is napping during the day helps, as does having a partner or family member who can assist with household chores.

Q Should I worry if I'm not getting enough sleep?

Don't be hard on yourself—pregnancy and the first 6 months with a new baby is extremely demanding physically and emotionally, and just getting through the day is an achievement in itself. If you have "baby blues" or if you feel depressed, seek professional advice. Depression can negatively affect infant-mother bonding as well as your own state of well-being.

Sleep and menopause

Does sleep quality change with menopause?

During menopause, many women are less satisfied with their sleep than previously. The most common complaint is difficulty falling asleep. Other problems include an increase in night-time awakenings and daytime drowsiness. However, actual sleep time and sleep stages are not different from those in premenopausal women, so differences in perception of poor-quality sleep probably have a more subtle background.

Are all sleep and health problems in menopause related to changes in hormone levels?

Many women assume that symptoms such as weight gain, sleep disturbances, and fatigue are related to hormonal changes alone, but this is a misconception that can lead to women missing potentially reversible and treatable causes of poor health. Postmenopausal women are at increased risk of snoring and sleep-disordered breathing, which can be the cause of daytime sleepiness and fatigue. These conditions can be treated to improve the quality of life remarkably.

Why do I get hot flashes?

No one knows the precise mechanism of hot flashes or night sweats. Hot flashes can also occur in women receiving certain treatments for breast cancer. Hot flashes are worsened by smoking, excessive weight, and physical inactivity. They last about 3–5 minutes, but sometimes can go on for 20 minutes. Some women have up to 20 hot flashes a day; others 1–2 times a week. Hot flashes cause awakenings at night, and women report diminished sleep quality, but there is little evidence to show any major disruption to the various sleep stages.

Q What can I do about hot flashes affecting my sleep?

If the flashes are extremely disruptive, short-term hormone therapy (HT) is still the treatment of choice. However, many women are reluctant to try this due to the associated health risks. HT should not be used by anyone who has had breast cancer or a stroke. Antidepressants, such as selective serotonin reuptake inhibitors (SSRIs), or gabapentin may be useful.

MENOPAUSE

Menopause, the transition into midlife, is a normal event in every woman's life and most women live long enough to experience it. Generally, menopause is said to be present once there has been an absence of any menstruation for 12 months.

The average age at which menopause occurs in Western societies is 51.4 years but it can occur between 40 to 58 years and is also influenced by lifestyle and genetic factors such as smoking, obesity, ethnicity, oral contraceptive use, age at menarche, and duration of breast-feeding. Some women can experience a very early menopause, in their thirties, and if the ovaries are removed at any age after puberty, menopause will result.

The time immediately before and after menopause is called the perimenopausal period. It is a period of transition where changes take place in the hormonal system and brain (with the decreasing production of estrogen and progesterone). Sleep disturbances and daytime fatigue are the most commonly reported symptoms during menopause. Other symptoms include hot flashes, mood disorders, and night sweats.

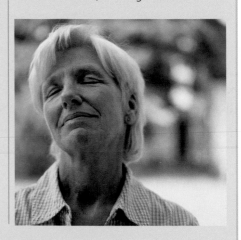

Can alternative therapies help with hot flashes?

The evidence for complementary and alternative therapies is not strong and their effectiveness is questionable. It might be worth trying acupuncture, yoga, or herbal treatments containing phytoestrogens such as red clover, soy, dong quai, or black cohosh. Obviously a cooler bedroom environment is better than a warm or hot one. The strategies outlined on pp28–34 may also help stem development of insomnia and ingrained bad habits.

How does stress during menopause affect sleep?

As estrogen levels decline, the heart and blood vessels as well as other hormones become more sensitive to stress. Increasingly, there is evidence that even day-to day hassles can impact sleep more significantly during menopause and result in frequent awakenings, less sleep time and slow wave sleep, and poorer quality sleep overall. It is therefore important to try and minimize stress in your life.

Are there any particular sleep disorders associated with menopause?

Obesity, raised blood pressure (hypertension), and sleep apnea are more common after menopause. Increases in weight can't be blamed just on menopause; they are more likely to be the result of normal aging and reduction in physical activity. Obesity is a risk factor for sleep apnea

Are there any other medical illnesses that are more common after menopause and that can disrupt sleep?

Depression and mood disorders become more common after menopause and can result in sleep disruption. Undergoing a hysterectomy after menopause can worsen symptoms of menopause and lead to mood problems. Cancer becomes more common after this stage in life as well and has its own problems associated with diagnosis and management. The incidence of thyroid problems increases and is more common in women; hypothyroidism is associated with fatigue.

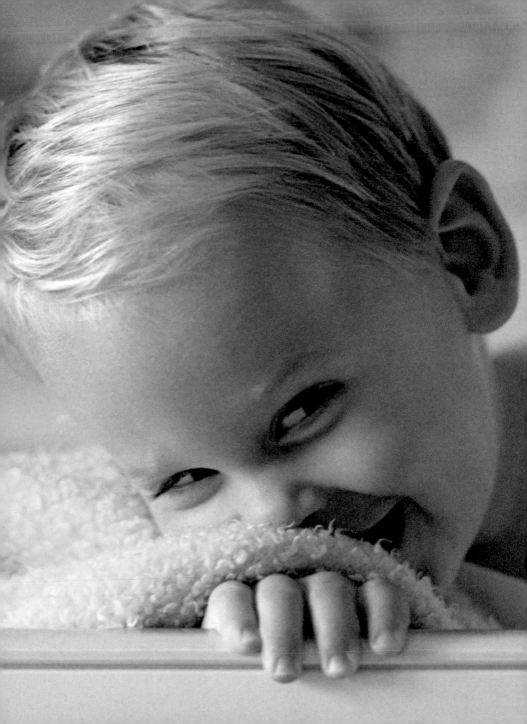

Children and adolescents

Sleep is crucial to the mental and physical development of children, who need to spend about 40 percent of their time sleeping. Their sleep requirements vary as they grow. Children are often exposed to "sleep stealers," such as caffeine, television, the Internet, and other activities that may result in sleep disruption. They can suffer the same sorts of sleep disorders as adults, so you should discuss any concerns with their pediatrician.

Babies

Q How much sleep do newborn babies need?

Sleep for the first 1–2 months of life usually occurs around the clock. The sleep-wake cycle comprises sleep and waking to be fed, changed, or nurtured. Newborns have an irregular sleep-wake cycle and sleep anywhere from 10 to 18 hours a day. Wake times can last from 1–3 hours at a time. Sleep is very active and half of a baby's sleep time is spent in REM sleep (active sleep).

Q How can I help my baby develop a sleep pattern?

Newborns should be put to bed when they are sleepy so they will start to learn how to get themselves to sleep. There are many theories and many books on how to develop sleep patterns in newborns and infants, but each child will have his or her own pattern that can gradually be adapted to our society's day–night cycle. Exposure to bright light and play during the day will keep a baby awake for longer, while a quieter and dimmer environment toward nightfall will be more conducive to sleep.

Q Does a breastfed child develop sleep disturbances after breast-feeding stops?

There is currently no evidence to suggest that breast-feeding your child (which involves a lot of awake time during the night) will lead to sleep disturbances once the child comes off the breast.

Q How should a baby be put to bed?

Babies should be put to bed when they become sleepy, and not when they are asleep. Make sure the head, face, and neck are clear of bedclothes and put the baby on his or her back. (See also box on SIDS, p149.)

Is co-sleeping good or bad for babies?

Co-sleeping (sharing a bed) is common in many cultures. There is no hard and fast evidence to suggest an increased risk of suffocation of the child. It is generally recommended that the infant be put to sleep in a separate room from the caregiver to avoid affecting the sleep-wake cycle of the adult. Many parents feel they are thereby becoming inattentive to their child's needs, but there is some evidence to suggest that they tend to get up even more often if they hear the child crying. There is some evidence to suggest that children who later develop sleep problems experienced co-sleeping in their infancy. In adults, sleeping apart has been shown to lead to a more refreshing night's sleep.

How does colic in my baby affect his/her sleep?

Colic is one of the more common disorders affecting sleep in infants. Usually it ends by 4 to 5 months of age. It is characterized by fussiness that is inconsolable in the late afternoon or evening hours. It is thought that colic reflects development of the brain during the first few months of life. Eventually the colicky behavior will settle, but associated sleep problems may not unless the parents or caregivers enforce a sleep-wake routine consistently. Colicky infants miss periods of sleep during their attacks, which can affect their sleep-wake cycle.

Once the colic has ended, how do I get my baby to sleep?

You must enforce regular daytime and night-time sleep patterns and adhere to them. The morning wake-up time is the most important aspect of the schedule—it must be fixed and consistent. Bedtimes at night should also be strictly adhered to. Being persistent with this routine is the single most important aspect of getting your baby back into a regular pattern.

Q Can cow's milk allergy cause problems with sleep in infants?

It can be difficult to differentiate cow's milk allergy from colic. However, your doctor will be able to do some blood tests to establish the diagnosis of allergy. Infants with cow's milk allergy often have very frequent night-time awakenings and their total sleep time is reduced. Crying during the daytime is common and the infant appears to be fussy. Problems with behavior and sleep can be easily resolved once cow's milk-based formula is discontinued. Symptoms should normalize within about 2 weeks.

Q My baby needs to drink a lot during the night—is this affecting her/his sleep?

Excessive nocturnal fluid intake is a recognized cause of disturbed sleep at night both for the baby and parents. Babies who drink large volumes of fluid (8–32oz) during the night typically awaken with heavily soaked diapers in the morning. From the seventh month, the infant should not be waking up at night to feed. Reasons for awakening to eat at night include: a learned response associating food with sleep, bladder distension causing awakening, and learned hunger. If large volumes of fluid are consumed the problem is one of excessive fluid intake. If the infant consumes small volumes of fluid, then the association of sleep with the presence of a parent is more important.

Q How can I wean my baby off fluids?

The trick is to gradually reduce the amount of the nightly feeding and fluid during the night over a period of about 1–2 weeks. Diluting milk with water can also help. If you are breast-feeding and your baby's cry results in "letting down" of milk, it may be better for you to express this milk and feed it through a bottle, diluting it gradually and weaning your baby that way. Your letdown will stop once the baby is sleeping through the night and no longer wakes up crying.

SLEEP AND SUDDEN INFANT DEATH SYNDROME

Sudden infant death syndrome (SIDS), or crib death, is the most common cause of death in children up to the age of one year. The diagnosis is made after all other possible causes of death have been excluded. Abnormalities in the breathing and heart rate responses during sleep are likely to contribute. The event that actually results in the death of a SIDS victim is a fall in blood pressure and slowing of the heartbeat until it comes to a standstill. Occasionally, there are genetic defects in the heart rhythm, which can also cause death in this manner.

RISK FACTORS

Other factors that may increase the risk of SIDS include smoking during pregnancy and after delivery. Probably the single biggest environmental factor that can be modified is smoking. Nicotine has even been found around the heart fluid in babies that have died of SIDS. Preterm babies, or those with a low birth weight or genetic problems in breathing control, are at risk. Other risk factors are illegal drug use by the mother during pregnancy, winter weather, and letting the baby sleep face down.

CARING FOR A SLEEPING BABY

Knowledge of these factors makes for some simple but effective strategies in caring for the sleeping baby. Always place the baby on his/her back to sleep. Avoid smoking and being around smokers during pregnancy and when the child is born. If your family has a history of heart rhythm abnormalities, it is important to tell your pediatrician so the baby can be carefully monitored and treated, if necessary.

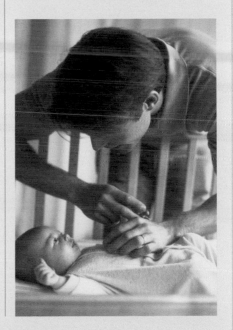

Myth "Children naturally develop an appropriate sleep-wake cycle"

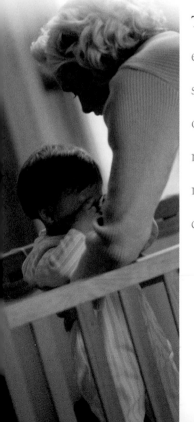

Truth This is not the case. The process of establishing a regular sleep-wake cycle in children should start right after birth. Children thrive on routine and their parents and caregivers must ensure that the bedtime and morning routine is enforced in a patient, persistent, and consistent manner.

From infancy to adolescence

How much sleep do infants need?

Infants between the ages of 3 and 11 months need a lot of sleep; in total, they should be sleeping about 14 to 18 hours a day. By the age of 6 months, most infants will not need to feed during the night and many will start sleeping through the night without waking up. About 4 in 5 infants should be sleeping through the night by the age of 9 months. The number of daytime naps that an infant will take ranges from 1 to 4 each day, and they are likely to last from 30 minutes to 2 hours at a time. The duration of night-time sleep should range between 9 and 12 hours a night.

Why should infants be put to bed while drowsy rather than when they're asleep?

Putting infants down while they are about to go to sleep will help them learn to fall asleep independently, and will also help them go back to sleep if they wake up, rather than being dependent on someone else to put them back to sleep.

My infant cries a lot when she wakes up during sleep—what could be causing that?

There are a number of reasons why an infant might cry during sleep. Is your child accustomed to you staying with him or her the whole time while he or she falls asleep? Has your child learned that each cry during sleep brings you running to the crib? Perhaps your child is going through a phase of separation anxiety (typically occuring between 8 and 9 months of age). Make sure that your child's daytime and night time routine is consistent and the sleeping environment conducive to sleep. Illness can also affect an infant's sleep patterns, so seek medical advice, if required.

Sleep hygiene for children

Children and adolescents need a well-planned routine. No child will ever hold it against you if you enforce a routine sleep-wake cycle. It is as important as all the other basic aspects of self-care (like appropriate toilet training, brushing teeth, and bathing). Sleep hygiene for children is very similar to sleep hygiene for adults except for a few extra considerations (see below).

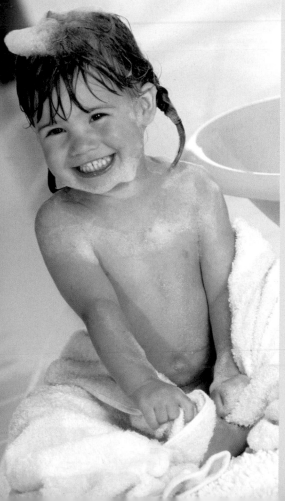

- Bedtimes should be consistent and predictible, while allowing for some flexibility, and should be firmly and consistently reinforced.

- As for adults, the child's bedroom should be kept quiet and dark during the night.

- The temperature in the bedroom should be comfortable (less than or equal to 75°F or 24°C).

- Try to minimize environmental noise. White noise may be helpful to mask a noisy environment.

- Children need to learn to fall asleep on their own. This means getting them to bed when they are drowsy but still awake so that they can learn to get themselves to sleep independently.

- Make sure that the environment is safe and secure and that the child feels this

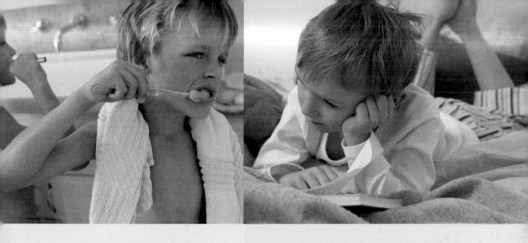

way about his or her bedroom. The child must be reassured that access to his or her parents is available if needed but not to help get to sleep.

- All vigorous activities should cease 1 to 2 hours before bedtime. If your child's bath-times provide too much excitement and stimulation at night, choose another time for bathing, such as late afternoon or in the morning.

- Avoid all products containing caffeine or alcohol. Note that references to the caffeine content may be hidden in the ingredient list in many types of food.

- If your child is hungry, give him or her a snack. Children should never be sent to bed hungry.

- Keep fluids before bedtime to a minimum and ensure that the child has been to the toilet before going to bed.

- Children should be allowed to protest and cry for a period of time that is appropriate for their age. Once the limit of protestation is reached, parents or caregivers can intervene and calm the child down. They should then leave the room while the child is awake and allow the child to fall asleep by him or herself. This process should continue until the child is asleep. It may take several hours to settle a child in this way, but if you are persistent and consistent, then the problem will settle quickly.

- Parents or caregivers should ensure that morning awakening times are consistent and strictly reinforced, because this is the most important part of the day in establishing a regular sleep-wake cycle.

- Daytime naps should be appropriate for the child's age and requirements. Naps should not be taken close to bedtime.

Q How much sleep do toddlers need?

Children between the ages of 1–3 years need about 12–14 hours of sleep in total during a 24-hour period. Naptimes during the day decrease with age and shouldn't be more than 1–3 hours in duration, the older the child gets. This is very much dependent on the sleep needs of the child in terms of development and genetically determined sleep needs that may already be apparent.

Q What kind of problems with sleep can occur at this age?

This can be a trying time for getting the child to sleep. It is a time in the developmental process where boundaries are being tested and children become more self-aware. There can be resistance to going to bed at night. Children are able to get out of bed by themselves and once their imagination starts to develop, nightmares and night terrors, as well as sleep-walking, can start to occur. It is therefore important that a routine is kept for sleep-wake times and reinforced as much as possible. Consistency is the key to success. Sometimes security objects (like a toy or a blanket) can be useful. If you have more than one child of this age in the household and they have different sleep patterns, it is often a good idea to have them sleep in separate rooms if at all possible.

Q How much sleep do preschoolers need?

After the age of 5 years, it is unusual for a child to require daytime naps. Children of this age still need a lot of sleep though—generally between 11 and 13 hours a night. Behavioral problems involving sleep can occur, with more awakening and opposition to bedtime. Once again, a consistent routine is the best way to counter this.

How much sleep do school-aged children need?

Between about 5 to 12 years of age, children have about the same sleep requirements as when they were preschoolers. Generally, 10 to 12 hours a night are needed to ensure maximum daytime functioning. At this period in their development, children experience many disruptions in their sleep patterns, such as extracurricular activities, engagement with computing and television, and less supervised intake of foods and drink which may contain caffeine (such as soft drinks). Disturbances to the sleep-wake cycle and inadequate sleep can lead to poor school performance, mood disorders, and hyperactivity. Many primary sleep disorders come to the fore during this time, including sleep apnea, narcolepsy, sleep-walking, and sleep-talking. A consistent bedtime routine is important.

How much sleep is enough during adolescence?

During adolescence, sleep requirements slightly fall, but are still more than in adults. Somewhere around 9 to 10 hours a night (especially in early adolescence) is necessary. However, there will be a lot of variation in this depending on genetically determined requirements.

What can disrupt the sleep of an adolescent?

Extracurricular and social activities and heavy homework schedules during adolescence take a toll on sleep. Many adolescents have independent access to computers and televisions in their own rooms that may deprive them of sleep. It is not unusual for adolescents to develop a phase shift in their sleep or for the first signs of delayed sleep phase syndrome (see p76) to occur. This can have a negative impact on school or job performance. A routine and consistent bedtime schedule is important during this phase of development, however hard it may be for parents to enforce it.

BEDTIME ROUTINES

Every family has its own routine and the one suggested below can be easily adapted to suit the way you interact with your children to get them to bed in as stressfree a manner as possible. It is important to be consistent as children thrive on routine. Being consistent also gives them a sense of security and purpose.

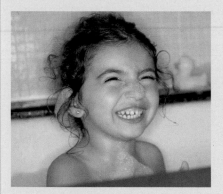

④ Dress in pyjamas after bath.

⑤ Quiet play or television in a room other than the bedroom for about 20–30 minutes. Your child should not have a television in his or her bedroom. Generally it is a good idea to watch something that is prerecorded so that if it is stopped, the program can be rewound and re-watched and your child knows that the next installment is still available.

① An early dinner.

② Quiet play after dinner—avoid computer games and other stimulating activities that might wind your child up or get him or her running around the house.

⑥ Brush teeth.

⑦ Go to the toilet.

⑧ Get into bed.

③ Bathtime with favorite toys about 1–3 hours before bed.

⑨ Short bedtime story.

⑩ Lights out.

Resist crying, calling out, and enreaties to read more or reenter the bedroom. Sometimes the child may take a while to settle, but he or she must learn to get to sleep by himself or herself.

Sleep problems in children

What sort of sleep problems do children get?

Children can experience the same sort of primary sleep disorders that adults do (see p50), although the prevalence of disorders is much lower. With the childhood obesity epidemic in Western countries, however, sleep apnea may become more common in children than previously. Medical illnesses and mood disorders that affect the child's health will also impact on sleep, just as they do in adults.

How can I tell if my child's sleeplessness is due to a medical disorder?

Most common conditions that disrupt sleep are due to pain, fever, and discomfort. One of the more common childhood illnesses is otitis media (an infection of the middle ear), which can cause sleep problems. The sleep disturbances come in the form of frequent and prolonged arousals at night and associated daytime sleepiness. A significant decrease in daytime activity can also occur. Prompt treatment results in prompt resolution of nocturnal symptoms. Nevertheless, it is important to maintain sleep hygiene (see pp132–133) and a regular sleep-wake schedule as much as possible during an illness. A child with a fever requires more sleep.

How is sleep affected in children with neurological disorders?

Disturbed sleep is often a feature of children who have problems with their nervous system or have either been born with or acquired an impairment of the senses, such as sight, hearing, and movement. Sleeplessness and night time awakening are frequent occurrences. Children with blindness and deafness may also experience significant disorders of the sleep-wake cycle.

How can I tell if my child has a sleep problem?

Always consider the possibility of a sleep problem if your child is sleepy during the day (this is abnormal for children who have a healthy balanced lifestyle), has started to show a decline in schoolwork or interest in activities, if his or her mood or activity levels have changed, or his or her behavior is becoming increasingly difficult or unpredictable. A simple way to remember the different causes of sleep problems is with the mnemonic "B.E.A.R.S."

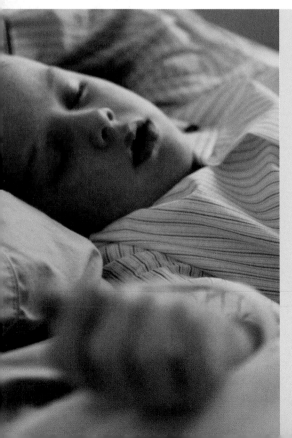

Ⓑ STANDS FOR BEDTIME PROBLEMS
- Does your child have difficulty getting to sleep?
- Does your child resist going to bed?
- Does your child take a long time to fall asleep?

Ⓔ STANDS FOR EXCESSIVE DAYTIME SLEEPINESS
- Is your child abnormally sleepy during the day?
- Does your child have great difficulty getting up in the morning?
- Does it take your child a while to get going in the mornings?
- Does your child fall asleep for no reason during the day?
- Does your child nap during the day (apart from developmentally appropriate naps)?

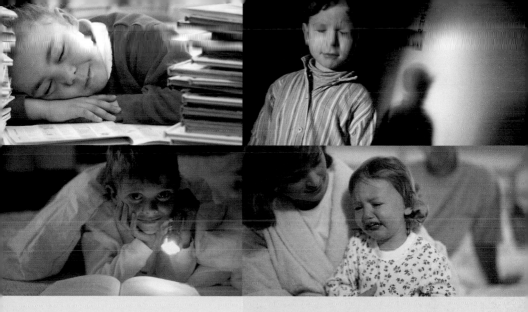

Ⓐ STANDS FOR AWAKENINGS AT NIGHT

- Does your child get up frequently during the night?
- Does your child stay up for long periods during the night?
- Does your child suffer from nightmares or night-time fears?
- Does your child sleepwalk regularly or wake up with night terrors?

Ⓡ STANDS FOR REGULARITY AND DURATION OF SLEEP

- How long does your child need to sleep?
- What is your child's sleep pattern like?
- Can your child follow a strict bedtime routine and get up at the same time every day?

Ⓢ STANDS FOR SNORING

- Does your child snore during sleep?
- Does your child have breathing pauses during sleep?
- Does your child get easily tired during the day or have behavioral problems, or has his or her school performance dropped off?

If you have answered yes to any of these questions (or if your child's sleep-wake routine is irregular) and you are concerned about your child's sleep or daytime function, please seek medical advice.

Q How are sleep disorders treated in children who have significant handicaps?

Sleep disorders in such children can be difficult to treat so it is best to seek professional help. You and your child may benefit from seeing a sleep specialist who may undertake investigations to assess how disturbed your child's sleep really is and whether there are any other concurrent disorders. It is also important to establish whether another medical disorder needs to be excluded before a diagnosis is made. Whatever the sleep disorder turns out to be, it can be treated by a variety of methods, as in adults.

Q Is attention deficit hyperactivity disorder a sleep problem?

Generally, parents of hyperactive children consider them to have more sleep disturbances than children who are not hyperactive. Children with attention deficit hyperactivity disorder tend to have more difficulty getting to bed and falling asleep, and are more restless sleepers, but there is some controversy over the issue of whether they have more disrupted sleep patterns than other children. Many hyperactive children also have frequent awakenings at night and increased restlessness. The occurrence of bed-wetting (see pp164–165) and sweating at night are more common compared to children without hyperactivity.

Q What are the characteristics of children with hyperactivity?

Children should be diagnosed as being hyperactive or having ADHD (attention deficit hyperactivity disorder) only by a specialist. Among the characteristics are a tendency to be fidgety and easily distracted, to disturb other children at school, to have difficulty concentrating and completing tasks, and to have rapid mood swings. Most children are restless and can become easily frustrated and rapidly destructive.

Can children with sleep apnea become hyperactive?

Yes. Children with significant sleep apnea will often behave in a very similar manner to children with ADHD. However, children with sleep apnea snore at night and there may be periods during the day when they are more sleepy than usual.

How should a child with hyperactivity be investigated?

As stated above, the diagnosis of ADHD should only be made by a specialist because it has many implications for the child and for the child's treatment. If sleep apnea is suspected, it must be investigated. There are many ways of managing hyperactivity including stimulants, counseling, and behavior modification (which can also be applicable to parents/caregivers). Once treatment is started, sleep problems tend to improve.

What are some of the more common childhood sleep disorders?

Children can suffer from primary sleep disorders just like adults do. The more common disorders that need to be considered in infants and toddlers have already been described. Other disorders include problems with limit-setting (often a parental problem), night-time fears, sleep-walking and sleep-talking, night terrors, bed-wetting (see pp164–165), snoring and sleep apnea, and disorders of circadian rhythms, especially in adolescence.

My child is frightened of going to bed— what can I do?

Night-time fears are very common in childhood. Children have active imaginations and may often experience vivid nightmares. Many fears occur as part of normal development, including fear of loss and separation from a parent/caregiver, sibling rivalry, and fear of death. These fears may be expressed through increased aggression, mood swings and moaning, and fear of sleeping alone or being left by the parent/caregiver at night.

Q How do I deal with fear in my child?

It depends on how long-standing and severe the problem is. If it has lasted a while and been difficult to manage, then you should consult a child psychologist. However, if you are aware of the fear developing and it has been present for a short while, your child may only need some understanding and firm support. Continue with bedtime rituals, but stay with your child a bit longer until he or she has settled, then withdraw. Changing the bedroom environment may make your child feel more secure.

Q Why is it such a struggle to get my child into bed every night?

You are probably giving in to your child's protests and have stopped being persistent and consistent with a bedtime routine and sleep hygiene measures. Rather than weathering the tantrums that will eventually subside anyway, you are reinforcing this protesting behavior and rewarding your child by giving in. Make sure you establish a bedtime routine and that other factors, such as the child sharing a bedroom with a brother or sister with different sleep requirements, is not undermining your efforts. You must stick to the regimen without fail, and be positive but firm. Consistency and persistence are important. Avoid becoming angry or threatening punishment because this leads to increased tension. You must decide who is going to win the bedtime struggle—you or your child?

Q What are night terrors?

In children, night terrors (*pavor nocturnus*) occur with the child suddenly awakening from slow wave sleep with a piercing scream or cry, accompanied by intense fear. The child might have a racing heart and feel sweaty. The attacks usually resolve by themselves. Night terrors occur regularly in 3 of 100 children, and occasionally in up to 15 in 100. They usually end during adolescence.

I find night terrors in my child very distressing—can they cause any harm?

Even though the sight of your child gripped by a night terror will upset you, try not to be distressed. The most important thing to remember is that, during a night terror, your child will not come to any harm and will not remember the event. Night terrors do not have any negative long-term consequences for your child's growth or development, nor are they a sign of any mood disorder or psychological problem.

Is there anything I can do when my child has night terrors?

Make sure that your child's sleeping environment is safe and that he or she cannot come to any major harm due to a fall from the bed. For example, it's not a good idea to let your child sleep on the top bunk if he or she sleep-walks or gets up during a night terror. Ensure a pleasant bedtime routine and consistent sleep-wake times for your child. If the problems are severe, occur very frequently, or don't seem to disappear as the child gets older, it is best to seek professional advice. Occasionally, medication will be useful and counseling may be necessary. You do not have to sit up all night by your child's bed. Gently guiding your child back to bed without awakening him or her is all that is necessary.

What is sleep-walking?

Sleep-walking consists of a series of complex behaviors that occur in slow wave sleep. Sleep-walking may stop spontaneously or the sleep-walker may return to bed. Falls and injuries may occur if walking leads to dangerous situations, such as out of a door and into the street or through a window. Sleep-walking occurs regularly in 1 to 3 in 100 children, and occasionally in up to 29 in 100 children. It will usually disappear after adolescence.

Bed-wetting

Bed-wetting during sleep is also called sleep-related enuresis. Enuresis is very common and at any one time millions of children suffer from it. Bed-wetting can be described as either primary or secondary. In primary enuresis, the child has never learned to control his/her bladder. In secondary enuresis, the child has at some stage been dry all night for at least 3 months.

Generally, enuresis should not be considered a significant problem under the age of 5 years if the child is developing and progressing normally. Approximately 3 in 10 four-year-olds have nocturnal enuresis, but only 1 in 10 six-year-olds, 3 in 100 12-year-olds, and 1 in 100 15-year-olds. Under the age of 11 years, boys are twice as likely to have problems as girls. There appears to be a familial predisposition: if a child has problems with nocturnal enuresis, there is a high chance that one or both parents had problems in childhood with enuresis as well.

WHAT CAUSES BED-WETTING?

The precise causes of sleep-related enuresis are not known. In primary enuresis, it is thought to be a problem with immaturity of the bladder and the systems in the body that relate to its control and the regulation of urine production. Primary enuresis will generally end with time and with the child's ongoing development. Secondary sleep-related enuresis is often associated with either the development of illness or with psychological factors. A urinary tract infection is one of the more common causes of secondary enuresis.

A urinary tract infection should be considered a possibility if there is wetting during the day as well as at night, abdominal pain, and burning or stinging when urinating. Other illnesses that can cause secondary enuresis include diabetes mellitus, kidney failure, and neurological problems relating to bladder control. Emotional problems commonly resulting in sleep-related enuresis include stress, family break-up and bereavement. If you are worried about your child's enuresis, then you must seek medical advice.

WHAT CAN I DO ABOUT MY CHILD'S BED-WETTING?

If your child has had a period of being dry and suddenly starts wetting the bed at night, you must seek medical advice. The bedwetting may be the result of psychological stress or the development of an illness.

If your child wets the bed even though she or he is old enough to stay dry, then the following tips might be useful:

• Make sure your child goes to the toilet before getting into bed.

• Restrict fluids an hour before going to bed—no final drinks before or while actually in bed.

• Wake your child during the night when he/she normally wets the bed and take your child to the toilet.

• Wearing diapers may be helpful.

• A bell-and-pad device is sometimes used. An alarm goes off whenever the pajamas or bed become wet. This is supposed to condition your child to wake up and feel the discomfort of being wet.

• Medication can be used but only if it is prescribed by your doctor. Medications commonly prescribed for enuresis include imipramine and desmopressin.

• Don't punish your child—he or she can't help it. Be sensitive and don't talk about the child's bed-wetting in front of others. Be patient with your child.

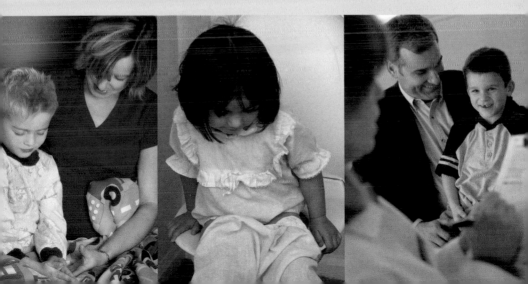

Q My child has started sleep-walking—is there anything I can do about it?

It is important to ensure that the environment is safe and that your child cannot walk through a window, plate glass door, or out of the house. You may need to install child-proof locks on doors or an alarm system on doors and windows. Don't let a sleep-walking child sleep on a top bunk. Try and ensure a regular sleep-wake schedule. In a child with frequent sleep-walking or who sleep-walks more often when distressed, medication and counseling may be appropriate. Guide your child gently back to bed; if you awaken the child, no harm will come to him or her.

Q My child is abnormally sleepy during the day—what could be causing this?

Reasons for being sleepy during the day include: not enough sleep at night due to frequent awakenings or an irregular sleep-wake regimen, an illness which is disrupting sleep and causing daytime sleepiness, circadian rhythm disorders, narcolepsy and other forms of daytime sleepiness (very rare), and sleep apnea.

Q How common is sleep apnea in childhood?

About 3 to 12 in 100 children snore regularly and, of these, about 1 to 3 in 100 have sleep apnea. Children with certain developmental disorders (such as Down syndrome) have an increased risk of sleep apnea. As obesity increases among children in our society, sleep apnea may become more common.

Q What are the consequences of sleep apnea in childhood?

Just as in adults, the consequences can be serious. These include adverse effects on the heart, blood vessels, and intellectual development, the latter leading to learning disabilities, behavioral problems (such as hyperactivity), and aggressive behavior. The repetitive dips in oxygen levels overnight in children with sleep apnea can have drastic and far-reaching effects on the developing brain.

How can I tell if my child has sleep apnea?

Loud snoring on a nightly basis is almost universally present in children with sleep apnea. The snoring is accompanied by labored breathing, breathing pauses, and choking noises. Sometimes, children with sleep apnea will wet the bed, experience sweating at night, and wake up with a dry mouth in the morning. Children are not often sleepy during the day, unlike adults, so attention must be paid to other indicators such as poor school performance, aggressive behavior, hyperactivity and morning headaches. If sleep apnea is very severe, a child can have failure to thrive. As in adults, the best way to diagnose sleep apnea is by doing an overnight sleep study. If you suspect that your child has sleep apnea, you must discuss this with your doctor and seek referral to a specialist for assessment.

How is sleep apnea treated in children?

The most common causes of sleep apnea in normal children are related to structural problems with the face or jaw, or to large tonsils and adenoids. Tonsillectomy and adenoidectomy are the first-line treatment for sleep apnea in children and are relatively simple surgical procedures to perform. However, they must be performed only after a specialist has fully investigated the child's sleep disordered breathing at night. Surgery to the jaw (if it is very small) or orthodontic treatment may be necessary in a small number of children with sleep apnea. CPAP treatment is also used (see pp62–63). Children who are obese must lose weight.

My child snores— is this OK?

Recent evidence suggests that children who snore have increased respiratory effort with the snoring. This may have adverse effects on behavior and intellectual functioning. If you are concerned about your child's snoring, especially if it is loud, disruptive, and habitual, consult your doctor.

PRESCRIBED MEDICATIONS FOR CHILDREN WITH SLEEP DISORDERS

Generally, most problems with sleep in childhood can be effectively addressed using behavioral techniques such as implementing a bedtime routine and ensuring that a regular sleep-wake schedule is consistently adhered to. This means that parents have to take responsibility and show some discipline themselves. However, depending on the disorder and its severity, medications can sometimes be prescribed. Some of the medications that might be prescribed in the treatment of childhood sleep disorders are listed in the table below.

SLEEP PROBLEM	MEDICATION	DRUG CLASS
Sedation	Diphenhydramine	Antihistamine
Enuresis; depression	Imipramine	Tricyclic antidepressant
Enuresis	Desmopressin	Hormone (ADH) analog
Parasomnias; seizures	Clonazepam	Benzodiazepine
Sedation	Lorazepam	Benzodiazepine
Sedation; phase advance	Melatonin	Hormone
Sedation	Zaleplon	Nonbenzodiazepine
Sedation	Zolpidem	Nonbenzodiazepine
Narcolepsy	Dexamphetamine	Stimulant
Narcolepsy; ADHD	Methylphenidate	Stimulant
Cataplexy	Clomipramine	Tricyclic antidepressant

Adolescent sleep-wake patterns

Q My 15-year-old boy stays up until late and can't get up in the mornings—is he just a "night owl"?

Perhaps. However, social and environmental factors can cause adolescents to shift the phase of their sleep-wake pattern. Factors that can contribute to this shift include a full extracurricular program (lots of homework as well as afterschool activities), a busy social life, a television and computer in the bedroom that can be used till late, poor adherence to a regular sleep-wake schedule, or parents who have difficulty with limit-setting. Of course, there may be a genetic determinant to staying up late, but this must be distinguished from behaviors that have led to the exacerbation or development of this tendency.

Q When does staying up late into the night become a problem?

Staying up late and going to bed late becomes a problem if it starts interfering with daytime functioning. If an adolescent has difficulty sleeping at a normal time, and because sleep needs are still high (9–10 hours a night), he or she might find it difficult to get up in the morning. If this means being late for school, missing the first class, or falling asleep in class, your adolescent has a problem.

Q Could my 15-year-old have delayed sleep phase syndrome (DSPS)?

Most often, the answer is "no" and the phase shift is due to behavioral reasons, such as an overloaded activity and school schedule, social activities, or work schedule. There must also be an absence of any mood or medical disorder. DSPS is a circadian rhythm disorder with an exaggerated "night owl" pattern of sleep and wakefulness.

Q How will I know whether my teen has DSPS?

Generally, the adolescent with delayed sleep phase syndrome (DSPS) has sleep onset and waking times that are delayed by 3–6 hours when compared to conventional sleep-wake times. The disorder should be present for one month or longer and other possible reasons for daytime sleepiness should be discounted. If your adolescent does have DSPS, he is likely to be sleepy and ready to go to bed between 2am and 6am and will generally get up some time between 10am and 1pm. You can expect his sleep to be normal. He will normally not be hungry in the mornings and will tend to want to eat closer to bedtime. If allowed to sleep late, he will also feel better and report less daytime sleepiness, especially on weekends and holidays.

Q How can I help my 15-year-old son to get back into a more normal pattern of sleeping and waking?

The most important thing for you to do is to evaluate not only your 15-year-old's lifestyle but also the way in which you help—or don't help—reinforce a consistent sleep-wake schedule. Look at his activities both at school and after school, and note down the times at which they occur. Try to schedule activities for earlier parts of the day or reschedule them outside the school week. Sleep hygiene is still incredibly important at this age, just as it is at any other. It is extremely important to establish a consistent bedtime and, crucially, a getting-up time for the mornings. Together, these will help train his circadian rhythm. Televisions have no place in the bedroom, where they are a common distraction for adolescents, and they should be removed and placed elsewhere in the home; if possible, computers should also be moved out of the bedroom. Encourage your teen to avoid caffeinated drinks, including caffeine-containing soft drinks, late at night.

What about bright light therapy for DSPS?

Apart from the common-sense measures discussed before, bright light therapy can be very useful. Bright light exposure should be scheduled for early in the morning. Strong light after sunset should be avoided. Remove coverings and dark curtains from windows and place the bed where the most direct sunlight will be present. An east-facing or south-facing bedroom will increase morning light exposure. In the winter, a lightbox may be very effective and generally a box that emits 10,000 lux will be sufficient (a lux is a measurement of light intensity). Light exposure is more effective if combined with exercise. Avoid light after sunset as much as possible. Even the glare from a computer screen may be sufficient to phase delay someone. As the morning exposure to light is introduced, the time of going to bed generally advances.

Are there any other forms for treatment apart from bright light therapy?

Melatonin can be useful for the treatment of DSPS—discuss the dose with your doctor. Occasionally, advancing bedtime one hour at a time, until the appropriate bedtime has been reached, can be tried. This should only be done during a period when school and other activities will not be affected. Guidance from a health professional is ideal.

How can a new sleep-wake schedule be maintained?

Once the DSPS has been controlled, a strategy must be put in place by the family to try and counter any instances which may put the adolescent back into his old sleeping patterns. Danger times for this are weekends and school vacations, when a few late nights followed by sleeping late will put everything back to where it started.

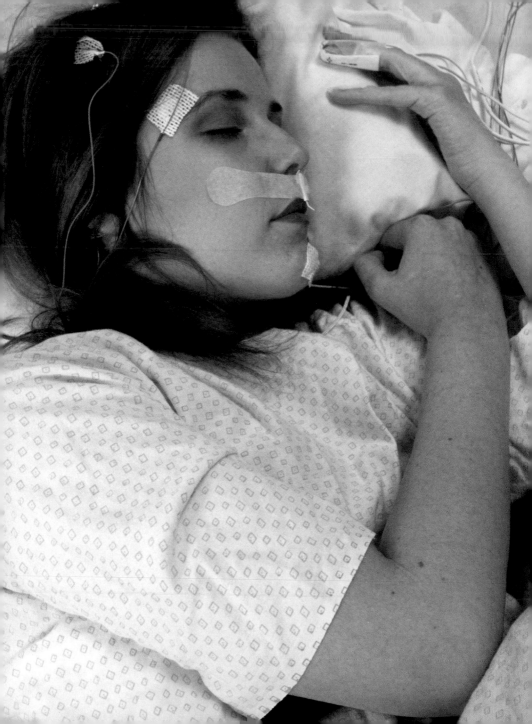

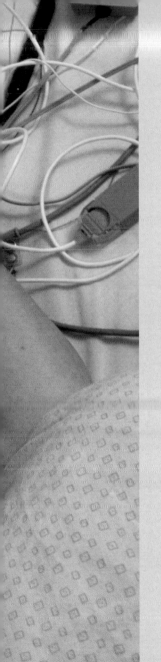

Tests and treatments

You may have picked up this book because you have problems with sleep; maybe your partner, friend, colleague, child, or a relative has sleep problems. Do you really have a sleep problem? How do you get a sleep problem investigated? What kinds of tests are done to diagnose sleep disorders? What are the treatments? This chapter gives you a brief outline of answers to questions like these.

Investigating sleep problems

Q How do I discuss a sleep problem with my doctor?

Doctors nowadays are much more aware of sleep problems and realize how important sleep is to health and normal functioning. Discussing a sleep problem with your doctor should be as natural as discussing a cough. If the problem is simple, then, often, your doctor will be able to guide you in examining your lifestyle and issues concerning sleep. If the problem is more complicated, you may be referred to a specialist in sleep medicine.

Q How are sleep problems investigated?

There are many ways to investigate sleep problems. People with insomnia are best served by first addressing sleep hygiene issues, or, if there is significant mood disturbance, to a psychiatrist or counselor, who can help uncover the reasons for the sleep disorder. People with chronic pain may benefit from referral to a specialized pain clinic that uses a multidisciplinary approach. Children with sleep disturbance should be referred to a pediatrician or a sleep specialist with experience in pediatrics.

Q Where are sleep disorders investigated?

This depends on the type of sleep disorder you might have. If sleep apnea is suspected, you might be referred for an overnight study at a sleep center (sleep lab) or even be sent home with recording equipment that you return to the sleep center the next day. If narcolepsy is suspected, you should be investigated in a sleep center where they can also conduct tests of daytime sleepiness.

ASSESSING YOUR OWN SLEEP

You are best placed to know what your sleep is like. To examine the patterns and quality of your sleep, you can ask yourself the following questions. These questions are modeled on the Pittsburgh Sleep Quality Index, which is designed to assess sleep in adults.

① When do you usually go to bed?

② How long do you usually take to fall asleep?

③ When do you usually get out of bed in the morning?

④ How many hours of actual sleep do you get on an average night (this does not refer to the actual number of hours you spend in bed)?

⑤ How often do you have trouble sleeping because of:
- Being unable to get to sleep within 30 minutes of getting into bed?
- Waking up in the middle of the night or early morning?
- Getting up to go to the toilet during the night?
- Inability to breathe comfortably?
- Coughing or snoring loudly?
- Feeling too cold?
- Feeling too hot?
- Experiencing bad dreams?
- Being in pain?
- Other reasons?

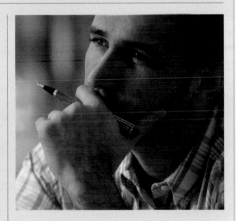

⑥ Do you often take medicine to help you get to sleep?

⑦ How often do you have trouble staying awake while driving, taking part in social activities, or during meals?

⑧ How difficult is it for you to keep up your enthusiasm to get things done?

These questions are designed to make you think about your sleep patterns and overall sleep. If you are concerned about any of your responses, you should seek medical advice.

Q **What kinds of sleep investigations are there?**

Sleep investigations take many forms and are adapted to the wide variety of disorders that are diagnosed by sleep specialists and respiratory specialists. Some investigations must be done in a sleep center; others can be done in the comfort of your own home. The main sleep-related investigations that are performed in a sleep center include polysomnography; multiple sleep latency testing and maintenance of wakefulness tests; and tests of vigilance. Monitoring of sleep using portable systems, actigraphy, keeping a sleep diary, and filling out questionnaires about your sleeping habits can all be done at home.

Q **What is polysomnography?**

The most common investigation in a sleep laboratory is polysomnography (PSG), which is described on p14. PSG allows the sleep specialist to assess how much you have slept and what the quality of your sleep was. At the same time, information is obtained on your breathing patterns during sleep and on any abnormal movements during sleep such as periodic limb movements.

Q **What does polysomnography involve?**

Polysomnography involves an overnight stay in a sleep center. This investigation is not as daunting as it sounds. The laboratory is usually set up to look like a bedroom. Each person sleeps in his or her individual bedroom, which is also sound-proofed. Nurses or technicians are present all night and keep a close eye on participants so that problems, if any, can be dealt with immediately. In the morning, you can leave the lab and get on with your day normally, just as if you had spent a night sleeping in your own home.

Are there investigations that can be done without going into a sleep center?	Although most sleep specialists do not recommend home studies, some centers lend portable recording devices for overnight use. The patient puts the device on at home and return it the next day. The overnight information stored on a computer chip in the device is downloaded and interpreted by a sleep technologist or sleep physician. The devices range from sophisticated machines to simple oximeters that are minimally obtrusive. Some centers use minimally invasive devices with video recording during the night to diagnose certain sleep disorders.
What is a multiple sleep latency test (MSLT)?	This is a daytime test of sleepiness and should ideally follow an overnight PSG in the sleep center. The patient is asked to have naps on 4–5 separate occasions several hours apart to assess whether there is excessive sleepiness during the day. This test is most commonly used to diagnose narcolepsy. The test is conducted in the sleep center and involves PSG. The data is recorded and assessed by the sleep technician and sleep specialist, who look for excessive sleepiness and note the time it takes the patient to fall asleep for each nap.
What is the maintenance of wakefulness test?	This tests assesses a person's ability to stay awake during the day. It comprises 3–4 periods evenly spaced across the day when the patient is asked to stay awake while inactive for a specified period of time. This test should ideally be preceded by an overnight PSG in the sleep center. The maintenance of wakefulness test is often used to assess the effectiveness of treatment for excessive daytime sleepiness, whatever the cause (obstructive sleep apnea, for example). As with MSLT, the test is done in the sleep center and involves PSG (see above and box on p14).

Q What is a test of daytime vigilance?

These are daytime tests that check one's ability to perform boring tasks that require significant concentration. They mimic, for instance, the level of attention required to monitor ships on a radar screen or to watch the road on a long drive. Examples include the Oxford sleep resistance (OSLER) and maintenance of wakefulness tests. These are performed in a sleep center; the results show whether significant sleepiness is present and affecting vigilance.

Q What is actigraphy?

Actigraphy is activity monitoring using a instrument which can detect motion. It helps differentiate periods of rest or sleep from periods of activity while awake. Actigraphy is commonly used to assess circadian rhythm disorders. Modern actigraphs are generally shaped like a wristwatch and worn on the ankle or wrist. The time you spend being inactive and active over 24 hours is downloaded from the actigraph and used to plot sleep and wake times in a more objective manner, as compared to a sleep diary.

Q What is a sleep diary?

A sleep diary is a simple tool for tracking sleep patterns and habits, and to document changes that occur with treatment (see pp46–47). Sleep diaries are especially useful in treating of circadian rhythm disorders, insomnia, narcolepsy, and where lifestyle issues are of concern.

Q Why are questionnaires used in the assessment of sleep problems?

Questionnaires such as those included in this book (see pp22–23, 57, 101–102) help you think about your sleep problem in a structured way. They also help researchers derive normal data for the general population against which an individual response can be assessed. They thus become important tools for a sleep professional to assess your problems and to monitor progress.

Treatments

How are sleep problems treated?

Throughout this book, each sleep problem has been dealt with in turn and specific treatments have been outlined. Treatments can include simple lifestyle changes, behavioral changes, talking therapies, medication, mechanical treatments, surgical treatments, dental treatments, light therapies, and complementary therapies. Sometimes a combination of several therapies is necessary.

What is meant by lifestyle changes?

Making lifestyle changes involves examining the daily patterns of your life and changing/modifying them if they are not producing the desired results. Lifestyle includes all the factors that make up your life and the way you run it, such as diet, exercise, sleep-wake routine, work, leisure, and relationships. Attention to each aspect of your lifestyle is beyond this book's scope but some aspects pertaining to sleep have been covered on p29.

What is meant by behavioral approaches to treating a sleep problem?

Behavioral techniques used to modify or change sleep behavior (usually in the treatment of insomnia) include sleep hygiene, relaxation exercises, and techniques for reducing recurrent and persistent thoughts during sleep. These include cognitive focusing, sleep restriction therapy, and systematic desensitization.

What is cognitive focusing?

This is the technique of focusing on pleasant thoughts and images when awakening at night. It is useful in the treatment of insomnia, especially in situations where the person wakes up during the night with negative thoughts that prevent him or her from getting back to sleep again.

Q What is sleep restriction therapy?

This is one treatment that can be of use in insomnia, when too much time is spent in bed but not enough of that time is spent asleep. People with this problem often end up going to bed early on some nights and late on others with the result that they end up with a very disrupted and inefficient sleeping pattern. The treatment involves reducing the amount of time spent in bed by an hour or more initially and going to bed at set times and getting up at set times. This helps consolidate sleep and strengthen circadian rhythms.

Q What is systematic desensitization?

This technique is very useful in people whose insomnia is related to anxiety and who associate negative thoughts with their bedtime routine. The person is asked to make a list of the negative thoughts and experiences associated with getting to sleep. The person then concentrates on associating pleasant ideas with the bedtime routine until it no longer becomes anxiety-inducing.

Q Which medications are commonly prescribed for sleep disorders?

The type of medication prescribed for your sleep disorder will differ depending on whether the problem is acute or chronic and whether it is potentially medication-responsive or not. There are many different classes of drugs that act on very different pathways in the brain. Probably the most commonly prescribed drugs are sedative drugs from the benzodiazepine and related classes. Some of the other drugs listed in the box on p181 are used exclusively for the treatment of excessive daytime sleepiness, such as modafinil, while others are used to treat a variety of disorders such as depression and anxiety (tricyclic antidepressants), and L dopa is used to treat Parkinson's disease as well.

COMMONLY PRESCRIBED MEDICATIONS FOR TREATING ADULT SLEEP DISORDERS

A large number of medications are used in the treatment of a variety of sleep disorders. They are listed below, but they must be prescribed by your doctor.

SLEEP PROBLEM	MEDICATION	DRUG CLASS
Cataplexy; depression	Imipramine	Tricyclic antidepressant
Enuresis	Desmopressin	Hormone (ADH) analog
Parasomnias; seizures	Clonazepam	Benzodiazepine
Sedation	Lorazepam	Benzodiazepine
Sedation; phase advance	Melatonin	Hormone
Sedation	Zaleplon	Nonbenzodiazepine
Sedation	Zolpidem	Nonbenzodiazepine
Sedation	Zopiclone	Nonbenzodiazepine
Sedation	Temazepam	Benzodiazepine
Narcolepsy	Modafinil	Stimulant
Narcolepsy	Dexamphetamine	Stimulant
Narcolepsy	Methylphenidate	Stimulant
Cataplexy	Clomipramine	Tricyclic antidepressant
Depression; cataplexy	Sertraline	Selective serotonin reuptake inhibitor (SSRI)
Depression; cataplexy	Fluoxetine	SSRI
Restless legs syndrome	Codeine	Opioid analgesic
REM-behavior disorder; Parkinson's disease	L-dopa	Dopamine agonist
Restless legs syndrome	Ropinirole	Dopamine agonist

Q **What does the term "talking therapies" encompass?**

Talking therapies involve counseling using techniques ranging from psychodynamic psychotherapy to cognitive-behavioral therapy (CBT). CBT is one of the most effective forms of psychotherapy, and deals specifically with issues that are causing problems in the patient's life such as self-esteem, anxiety, problems with coping, low mood, or self-defeating behavior. CBT involves the patient identifying the behavior, rating how he or she feels about it (anxious, stressed, depressed), and then challenging that feeling with rational thought. Once the feeling is challenged and more realistic alternative viewpoints are brought into play, the patient is then asked to again rate feelings again about coping with the situation.

Q **What is meant by mechanical treatments for sleep disorders?**

Mechanical treatment of sleep disorders encompasses the use of continuous positive airway pressure (CPAP) for sleep-disordered breathing or bilevel ventilation devices in patients with respiratory failure (see pp62–63).

Q **How applicable are dental and surgical treatments to sleep disorders?**

Surgery may help patients with sleep apnea who have a correctable facial, jaw, or tongue abnormality. Dental treatments for sleep apnea and snoring are mandibular repositioning devices or mouthguard devices that are fitted to the upper and lower jaws. Mouthguards are useful in the treatment of bruxism or tooth-grinding during sleep.

Q **How do I undertake light therapy?**

Light therapy is used to treat both circadian rhythm disorders and SAD (see pp104–109). It involves exposure to a lightbox at 10,000 lux for 30–60 minutes depending on the strength of light. Lightboxes can be bought easily, especially online. Further information can be obtained from the websites listed on p184.

Are complementary therapies effective in the treatment of sleep disorders?

Personal anecdotes suggest that herbal, homeopathic, and other complementary therapies such as reiki and hypnosis may be useful at times or even as adjuncts to other forms of therapy in the treatment of sleep problems. They are probably the most helpful when it comes to lifestyle problems involving the reduction of stress and anxiety levels. They may have a small role to play in dealing with insomnia. However, there is very little evidence from properly conducted trials on their true efficacy.

RELAXATION TECHNIQUES FOR GETTING TO SLEEP

There are many different relaxation techniques and you should choose one that suits you. Some people find meditation useful, while others enjoy yoga or tai chi. People with very high muscle tension may find it useful to do the progressive relaxation exercise first described by Edmund Jacobsen in 1983.

This exercise is intended to relax step-by-step all the different groups of muscles in the body. It involves lying on the floor on your back with legs uncrossed and out straight, and arms down by your sides. Your eyes should be closed. The exercises should last about 30–60 minutes, depending on the degree of muscle tension present, but can be abbreviated. Each muscle group in turn is tensed, then suddenly allowed to go limp, followed by relaxation for a couple of minutes. Start at your feet and gradually work up your body, tensing and relaxing each large muscle group in turn until you reach your head.

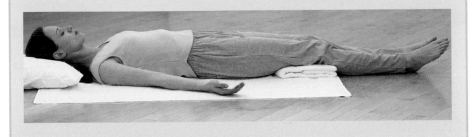

Useful addresses

American Insomnia Association
American Academy of Sleep Medicine
One Westbrook Corporate Center
Suite 920
Westchester, IL 60154
Tel: (708) 492-0930
Website: www.americaninsomnia
association.org

American Sleep Apnea Association
1424 K Street NW, Suite 302
Washington, DC 20005
Tel: (202) 293-3650
Website: www.sleepapnea.org

Awake In America, Inc.
PO Box 51601
Philadelphia, PA 19115
Tel: (215) 764-6568
Website: www.AwakeInAmerica.org

Canadian Sleep Society
Société Canadienne du Sommeil
Hôpital du Sacré-Cour de Montréal
Centre de Recherche, 3K
5400, boul. Gouin ouest
Montréal, QC H4J 1C4
Website: www.css.to

Children and Adults with
Attention Deficit / Hyperactivity
Disorder (CHADD)
8181 Professional Place, Suite 150
Landover, MD 20785
Tel: (301) 306-7070
Website: www.chadd.org

Narcolepsy Network
79 Main Street
North Kingstown, RI 02852
Tel: (888) 292-6522 / (401) 667-2523
Website: www.narcolepsynetwork.org

National Down Syndrome Society
666 Broadway, New York, NY 10012
Tel: (800) 221-4602
Website: www.ndss.org

National Sleep Foundation
1522 K Street, NW, Suite 500
Washington, DC 20005
Tel: (202) 347-3471
Website: www.sleepfoundation.org

Restless Legs Syndrome Foundation
819 Second Street SW
Rochester, MN 55902
Tel: (507) 287-6465
Website: www.rls.org

Index

About the Author

Renata L. Riha is a consultant in Sleep and General Medicine at the Royal Infirmary, Edinburgh, and an Honorary Senior Lecturer at the University of Edinburgh. Dr. Riha qualified in medicine at the University of Queensland and completed her training in respiratory and sleep medicine in Australia. She is a Fellow of the Royal Australasian College of Physicians and of the Royal College of Physicians of Edinburgh, and is active in the field of sleep research.

About the US Consultant

Anne Helena Remmes, MD obtained her medical degree from State University of New York at Stony Brook and is trained in internal medicine, neurology, and sleep medicine. She is a Fellow of the American Sleep Disorders Association and Director of Headache and Sleep Medicine at Columbia University of Physicians and Surgeons.

Author's acknowledgments

I would like to thank my family and friends, especially Dr. Heather Engleman, for their comments, and my colleagues at the Department of Sleep Medicine, Edinburgh, for their encouragement and for allowing the sleep diary to be reproduced.

For the publishers

DK Publishing would like to thank Ann Baggaley for editorial assistance; Isabel de Cordova and Kathryn Wilding for design assistance; and Jo Walton for picture research.

Credits

The publisher would like to thank the following for their kind permission to reproduce their photographs: (Key: a-above; b-below/bottom; c-center; f-far; l-left; r-right; t-top)

Alamy Images: Design Pics Inc. 165l; eStock Photo 73tr; Jennie Hart 165c; Martin Lladó//Gaia Moments 159tr; PHOTOTAKE Inc. 63; plainpicture GmbH & Co. KG 131cb; Purestock 139l; Stock Image/Pixland 136; Stockbyte Platinum 51, 66, 128; Stockbyte Silver 131b; **Corbis:** Paul Barton 116; Joe Bator 159cl; Dana Hoff/ Beateworks 33br; Kevin Dodge 112bl; FURGOLLE/Image Point FR 86; Rob Lewine 165r; Roy Morsch 7br; Jose Luis Pelaez, Inc. 131ca, 158; David Pollack 52; David Raymer 101; Norbert Schaefer 7bl, 111, 152; Anne-Marie Weber 142; Larry Williams 175; A. Inden/zefa 8; Ajax/zefa 112bc; G. Baden/zefa 30; Gulliver/zefa 36; Mika/zefa 20, 105bc, 122; Ole Graf/zefa 105fbl; Studio Wartenberg/zefa 33fbr; Tim O'Leary/zefa 7bc, 48; **Getty Images:** 82; Britt Erlanson 150; Flying Colours 6bl,

153l; Jason Hetherington 73tl; Jonah Light Photography 144; Jonathan Kirn 26; Yoav Levy 6bc, 172; Barbara Maurer 153r; Antonio Mo 46; Steven Peters 75; Andreas Pollock 33fbl; Martin Poole 159tl; Jake Fitzjones/Red Cover 33bl; Bill Robinson 156; Lauri Rotko 2; Alan Thornton 105fbr; Ross Whitaker 6br, 149, 159cr; Mel Yates 40; Yellow Dog Productions 29; **Masterfile:** Chad Johnston 138; **PunchStock:** 23r, 23l; **Images courtesy of Respironics. Inc. and its affiliates, Murrysville, PA:** 62fcl, 62cl, 62bl; **Science Photo Library:** BSIP Laurent 14; BSIP, Laurent/LAETICIA 107; Gusto 139r; Lea Paterson 131t; Cristina Pedrazzini 112br

All other images © Dorling Kindersley
For further information see: www.dkimages.com

Sleep hygiene tips pp152–153 adapted from *Principles & Practice of Pediatric Sleep Medicine*, Sheldon SH, Ferber R, Kryger MH, p133, © 2005, with permission from Elsevier.